Balancing the Chakras

Balancing the Chakras

by Maruti Seidman

North Atlantic Books
Berkeley, California

Balancing the Chakras

Published by
North Atlantic Books
P.O. Box 12327
Berkeley, California 94712

• • •

Cover, book design and illustrations in Chapter One © Carolina de Bartolo
Printed in the United States.

Balancing the Chakras is sponsored by the Society for the Study of Native Arts and Sciences, a nonprofit educational corporation whose goals are to develop an educational and cross-cultural perspective linking various scientific, social and artistic fields; to nurture a holistic view of the arts, sciences, humanities, and healing; and to publish and distribute literature on the relationship of mind, body, and nature. Printed in the United States of America.

This book is not intended to diagnose, prescribe, or treat any ailment, nor is it intended in any way as a replacement for medical consultation when needed. The author and publishers of this book do not guarantee the efficacy of any of the treatments and techniques herein described, and strongly suggest that at the first suspicion of any disease or disorder, the reader consult a physician.

Library of Congress Cataloging-in-Publication Data
Seidman, Maruti.
    Balancing the chakras / Maruti Seidman.
        p. cm.
    ISBN 1-55643-339-5 (alk. paper)
        1. Chakras. I. Title.
    RZ999 .S45 2000
    131--dc21   00-021574

1   2   3   4   5   6   7   8   9   /   04   03   02   01   00

This book is dedicated to my Spiritual Teacher,
Shri Dhyan Yogi Madhusudandasji who awakened the Universal
Love Energy within me.

Acknowledgements

There are many people who gave much of their time and creative
    energy in helping me complete this book:

Dhyan Yogi guided me to a place of peace within.
Paramanhansa Yogananda inspired me to write.
Ram and Sita gave me the courage to complete this book.
Hanuman gave me the perseverance to complete this book.
My son, Daniel, spent countless hours assisting me with my computer.
My daughter, Alana, inspired me to be creative.
Melinda Gladstone worked directly with me, editing and supervising
    the structure of this book.
Ahsha Hazen created the diagrams.

A special thanks to Rick Trace for all his wonderful help with the art-
    work, and to Liz Davidson for her editorial work.

A special thanks to Nicole George who worked directly with me in
    completing this project.

Finally, I would like to thank all the people of this planet who are
    living their lives immersed in love.

Contents

Chapter Three:
Healing and Transformation   69

Chapter Four:
Self Help for the Chakras   81

Chapter Five:
Chakra Healing through Meditation 143

Appendix One:
Symptoms and Imbalances
of the Chakras 157

Appendix Two:
Emotional Imbalances of the Chakras 167

Appendix Three:
Meditation Review 171

Bibliography 173

Diagrams

Oh Heavenly Mother

Oh Heavenly Mother
The Universal transformation awaits us
as our Planet Earth vibrates at its core.
We welcome the change, we honor the change,
and pray for guidance, eternal love, and union
with your spirit. We are blessed by your essence
and will always be humbly at your feet.
As the energy moves through the Universe,
So are we moved, like the wind passing
through a hillside on a cool Autumn day.
Transformation occurs every season, moving
and guiding us into a new awareness of who
we really are. Blessed is the change in nature
that activates our internal change. Blessed is
the opportunity that nature provides, helping
us move forward into the light. For where does
the light shine but from within? As we are
continuously affected by everything that
occurs outside, we forget about the light that
always glows inside. Awaken to your internal
beauty and honor the Cosmic Light of Love,
strength, and bliss—it is our natural birthright.
Just as the Heavenly Mother transforms the
Planet Earth through the seasons, she will
also transform us, when our light shines
on through.

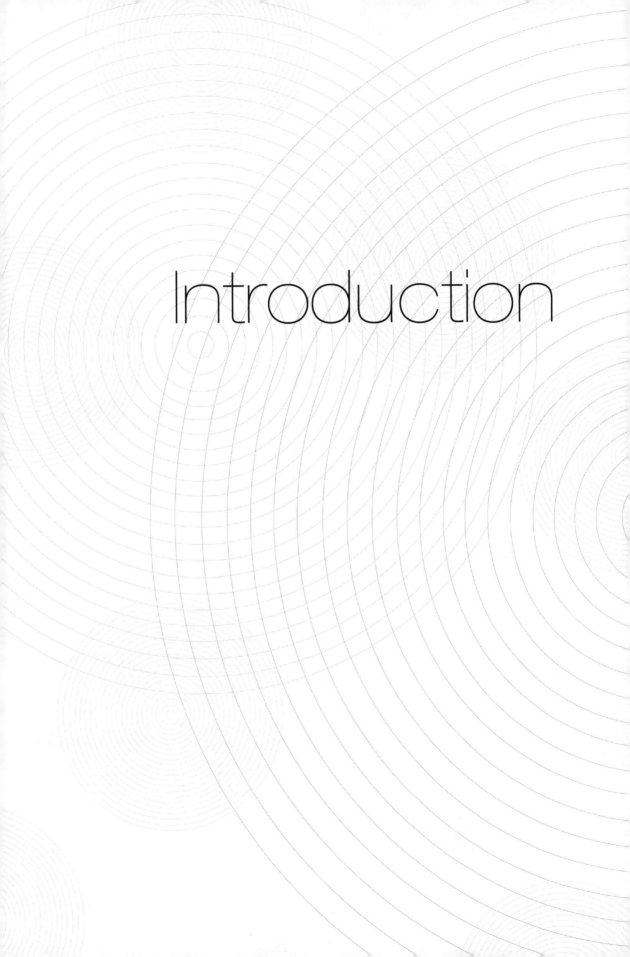

Introduction

ife is choice. The events and experiences that occur throughout a person's life constantly test her. People often respond to life's circumstances by creating thoughts and actions that swing them back and forth from high to low. Responding at the extremes creates stress and tension. The often overlooked response is the neutral response, a response that is balanced and in harmony with nature, the environment, and Spirit. The neutral response allows an individual to be centered and at peace in all situations.

When Spirit is honored through an individual's intuitive process, the daily choices of her life become grounded in the Universal Consciousness of God. Once connected to the God Energy, she can trust that the God Energy will guide and protect her throughout her life. This awareness reduces stress and tension, and allows her to be clear and free in all of life's situations.

People are blessed to have the Universal Consciousness of God at their fingertips, but blinded by their illusions of the physical world that keeps them from receiving these blessings. People are always seeking information and answers outside of themselves, not realizing that all their answers are within.

Working with the chakras is perhaps the easiest way for people to reconnect to their God Energy within. The chakra system of energy has been used for literally thousands of years by the Saints of the Far East as a means of helping people help themselves. Much of this information has been made available to the truth seekers in the West as an aid to healing themselves and all of mankind.

I sincerely hope this book helps you with your healing journey. If you have any questions about your healing process, or would like to attend one of my healing seminars, contact me at the telephone number or address at the beginning of this book. Om peace, peace, peace.

— Maruti Seidman
Autumn 2000 • Boulder, Colorado

Intro-
duction

Chapter One
The Chakras

The chakras are divine, subtle energy centers from which all experiences in life originate. They have been described as spinning vortices of subtle energy through which the individual receives, transmits, and processes the universal life-force energy. According to the saints and yogis of India, there are seven chakras located along the spine, each one interacting with the others. They form a subtle and psychic network of energy through which the body, mind, and spirit operate as one holistic system. The chakras are the subtle energy blueprint for the physical manifestation of the human form.

The sole purpose in gaining awareness of the chakra system is to assist the individual in achieving a state of harmony within her. When harmony is achieved, a person's consciousness can then weave the thread of love through her spiritual, mental, emotional, and physical beings. This will harmonize all her energies with the universal life-force energy.

Each chakra vibrates at a different rate of speed (some vibrate fast, some slowly), creating specific energy patterns associated with specific energy systems. The slower the vibrational rate of the chakra, the denser the form. The faster the vibrational rate of the chakra, the more intricate the form. For example, a chakra that vibrates at a slow rate of speed creates muscles and bones. A chakra that vibrates at a faster rate of speed creates the more complex nervous system. Though each chakra vibrates at a different rate of speed, this doesn't mean one chakra is better than another. Each chakra is a manifestation of divine energy, in a different form.

There are seven chakras along the front and back of the body (fig. 1). On the back, they are located along the spine, from the tip of the coccyx to the top of the head. On the front, they are located along the body's midline, from the tip of the coccyx to the top of the head.

The first chakra, located at the base of the spine (tip of the coccyx), creates the earth element. The earth element is moving at a very slow rate of speed. It creates structure and solid form in the body.

The second chakra, located in the pelvis, creates the water element. The water element is moving at a faster pace than the earth element, and wants to move like a stream flowing downhill into a lake. It creates movement throughout the body.

The third chakra, located at the navel center, creates the fire element. The fire element is moving at a faster pace than the water element and wants to expand. It creates warmth and heat as it moves upward and outward.

The fourth chakra, located at the chest, creates the air element. The air element is moving at a faster pace than the fire element, and wants to jump around from one stimulus to another. It creates constant motion.

The fifth chakra, located at the throat, creates the ether element. The ether element is moving at a faster pace than the air element, and wants to have room to move within the form. It creates space. Without space, there would be no form.

The sixth chakra, located in the center of the forehead, creates the mind's eye (third eye). The mind's eye is moving at a faster pace than the ether element, and is associated with pure spiritual energy. It represents knowledge of all things in the universe.

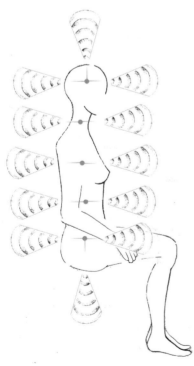

Figure 1

The seventh chakra, located at the top of the head, creates the thousand-petal lotus. The thousand-petal lotus is moving at a faster pace than the mind's eye, and is associated with complete union of spirit. It represents the total merging with universal love energy. All is one.

The seventh chakra, located on the top of the head, extends toward the sky as a cone-shaped funnel, expanding upward. The first chakra, located at the base of the spine (coccyx), extends toward the ground as a cone-shaped funnel, expanding downward. The second, third, fourth, fifth, and sixth chakras, extend outward from the center of the body (front and back), as cone-shaped funnels that widen.

Transformational Energy

All physical manifestations of energy find their source at the universal storehouse of energy, or the cosmic five elements. All matter contains the cosmic five elements of ether, air, fire, water, and earth. One gets a better understanding of this concept by examining the element of water. When the water element is in a solid state it is called ice. When ice forms, the earth element has manifested in water. As heat (fire element) is added to the ice, the ice turns to water, then steam. The steam is an expression of the air element. When the steam rises, it disappears into space. Space is a manifestation of the ether element. Thus, the cosmic five elements of ether, air, fire, water, and earth are present in one substance. Another example of the cosmic five elements manifesting in one form is in the qualities of different sounds produced by the human voice. A deep-rooted, heavily vibrating voice projects a feeling of solidity that corresponds to the earth element. As the voice becomes sweeter, the individual's creativity is enhanced, stimulating the water element. When the voice becomes intense, the fire element is stimulated. As the voice softens with gentleness and compassion, the air element is stimulated. Finally, the ether element gives the voice space from which to operate. Thus are the cosmic five elements of ether, air, fire, water, and earth present in sound.

The manifestation of divine energy is forever changing within the human body. It does not increase or decrease in strength, but continually changes form as it moves from one vibrational level to another, in accordance with the human body's needs. Do not lose sight of the universal law that states, "energy is energy." Energy is neither good or bad, it just is. Sometimes the human body needs more dense energy, and sometimes it needs lighter energy. It depends on what is going on within the individual at any given time. The human body creates more density or lightness in its vibrational field in accordance with its needs.

The Spinning Chakras

The chakras are vortices of subtle energy. Each chakra moves in a certain direction, in a spinning motion, either clockwise or counterclockwise. It is the spinning movement of the chakra that carries its divine messages to the energy systems of the body. Once the body receives the divine messages from the chakra, it acts accordingly to make corrections within its energetic systems to achieve balance and harmony (homeostasis).

The spinal system has its own unique electrical system that regulates the spinning of the chakras. On the right side of the spine, there is an electrical current with a positive charge. On the left side of the spine, there is an electrical current with a negative charge. In the central core of the spine there is an electrical current with a neutral charge. The positive electrical charge dominates the negative and neutral electrical charges. All three electrical currents begin at the tip of the coccyx, and travel upward to the top of the head. The right-side current travels up the right side of the spine until it comes to the top of the first chakra. It then splits. Part of the right-side current continues to travel up the right side of the spine and the other part crosses over the top of the first chakra to the left side of the spine at the bottom of the second chakra. It travels up the left side of the spine to the top of the second chakra, then crosses over to the right side of the spine at the bottom of the third chakra. The positive current continues to travel up the spine, looping around each chakra until it crosses over to the right side of the skull at the bottom of the seventh chakra, moves up the right side of the skull, and merges into the seventh chakra located at the top of the head. While the right side current is zigzagging along the spine to the seventh chakra, the left side current also is zigzagging along the spine to the seventh chakra. Together, they form a snake-like pattern (fig. 2). Since the right-side current is dominant, it spins the first chakra to the left as it comes up the right side of the first

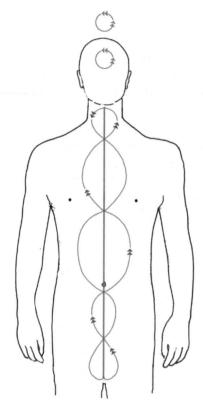

Figure 2

chakra and crosses over to the left side of the spine at the bottom of the second chakra. This creates a counter-clockwise motion for the first chakra. When the right-side current crosses over to the right side of the spine at the top of the second chakra, it spins the second chakra to the right. This creates a clockwise motion for the second chakra. In this way, the chakras spin in alternating ways. The first chakra spins counter-clockwise, the second chakra spins clockwise, the third chakra spins counter-clockwise, the fourth chakra spins clock, wise, the fifth chakra spins counter-clockwise, the sixth chakra spins clockwise, and the seventh chakra spins counter-clockwise.

Kundalini Energy

Kundalini is the Sanskrit word (Sanskrit is the ancient holy language of India) used to describe the divine energy that exists in every human being. It is the spark of life, the creative universal force that manifests an individual's life form. Without kundalini energy, life would not exist.

When the male and female energies unite in the womb at the time of conception, the seed power of creating a human being is activated and miraculously creates the blueprint for the human form. As vortices of kundalini energy begin to move in the womb, the chakras are formed. The chakras interpret and assimilate the kundalini energy, creating the human body. When the task is complete, a new life emerges from the womb as a newborn baby. Many people believe that babies are helpless and completely dependent upon their parents for survival. Nothing could be further from the truth. Newborn babies are the completed products of life's miracle and they come into this world as whole, complete, spiritual, God-children. They are completely functional and ready to assimilate their earthly experiences. Babies are really teachers and show the way of unconditional love, unattachment to ego, and how to be blissful in every moment. What a blessing babies are!

Once the human body is formed in the womb, kundalini energy concentrates into the first chakra. The body automatically places a psychic lid over the first chakra, keeping the kundalini energy intact. Some people say that kundalini energy sleeps in the first chakra. This is not true. Kundalini energy is in perpetual motion, going round and round in a counter-clockwise motion within the confines of the first chakra. There is always a small amount of kundalini energy that is released from the first chakra. Without this small amount of kundalini energy flowing through the body, the body could not function.

With the energetic blueprint completed, life goes on. The human being then enters into the cycles of life and death, many, many times. Hopefully, with each rebirth, the individual will begin to understand the purpose of life, and work toward the goals of self-realization, then God-realization. Once God-realization occurs, there is no more need to be reborn in human form. Individual souls can then move on to the astral plane. The astral plane is etheric. One needs only to think a thought, and it becomes true. If he wants a certain tree to produce a papaya, he just thinks it and the tree automatically produces the fruit. However, there are also many life lessons to be learned on the astral plane, and the individual can remain on the astral plane until he completely gives up all his attachments and desires. Once he has completed all astral-plane life lessons, he is ready to move on to the causal plane. The causal plane is even more etheric than the astral plane. There is no form at all on the causal plane, just ideas and concepts. Once the individual has completed all the life lessons on the causal plane, there is complete merging with the universal energy, and all is one.

The life and death cycle that humans experience is quite a process. Paramanhansa Yogananda (an enlightened saint from India) says it could take up to one million years of good, natural living for a human being to work through all his earthly lessons and move on to the astral plane. Yogananda also says that the longest time in between human incarnations is about five thousand years. That means at least two hundred lifetimes, or many, many more, to complete life lessons—quite a long time. However, there is a much quicker way to complete life lessons and set the soul free, within several lifetimes. This process is accomplished through the conscious reactivation of the kundalini energy in the first chakra. Once kundalini energy is consciously reactivated, it moves up through the chakra system until it merges with the seventh chakra located at the top of the head. As kundalini energy moves upward through the chakras, the chakras are purified one by one, until the entire chakra system is cleansed. This can take quite some time because each chakra has stored-up spiritual, mental, emotional, and physical issues that must be cleared before kundalini energy can progress up to the next chakra. As each chakra is being healed, an individual can be faced with many challenges and lessons that correspond directly with that chakra. Once all the chakras are healed, kundalini energy can then merge with the seventh chakra, bringing great spiritual awareness to the individual. Once kundalini energy can be consciously held in the seventh chakra, enlightenment occurs. There is no longer a need for the soul to be in the human body, and a person can consciously leave the human body whenever he chooses to.

The conscious reactivation of kundalini energy can occur by the grace of an enlightened master. This is usually accomplished in a ceremony or ritual that an enlightened master performs with the student. Both the master and the student have to be in consent before the ritual is performed. During the ritual, the enlightened master consciously transfers some of his divine energy to the student, reawakening the student's kundalini energy, after which, the enlightened master and student remain in relationship for the rest of their lives. Even if the enlightened master leaves his body, he can still guide the student on the intuitive and psychic planes. If the student is sincere and listens to all of the instructions from the enlightened master, the student can become enlightened in her lifetime too. Even if the student falls short of the goal and does not reach enlightenment, she is often born with a high spiritual awareness during the next lifetime, allowing her to continue her spiritual journey. Sometimes, the enlightened master will follow the student's soul into the next lifetime, reconnect with her, and initiate (activate the kundalini energy) her once again. This shows how much love the enlightened master has for his students and how determined he is to assist his students in reaching their goals of God-realization.

When an enlightened master transfers his divine energy to his student during the ritual, the exchange is so powerful that all the negative *karma* (karma is a person's actions in all her lifetimes) of the student can be completely cleansed and purified. It doesn't matter what the issues are, or how many lifetimes ago the karma originated; all can be cleansed. This frees up the student's energy so she can make new choices and progress rapidly toward the goal of self-realization. The enlightened master will always remain bonded with the student. It is the most important relationship the student will ever have in her lifetime. A person's parents give her a physical body; however, the enlightened master cleanses her soul and prepares her for union with God. Any individual who has the grace and good fortune of meeting an enlightened master and entering into the student/master relationship will have really good karma. That person is also incredibly lucky.

If kundalini energy is reactivated without the guidance of an enlightened master, it could present many difficulties for an individual. A surge of unguided kundalini energy running through the body could completely overwhelm the individual. Paramanhansa Yogananda said that if a person was not ready to receive the reactivated kundalini energy, the effect would be similar to putting a fifty-watt bulb into a million-watt circuit of energy—the bulb would obviously explode. The effect of having kundalini energy reactivated without the guidance of the enlightened master could be devastating; resulting in many spiritual, emotional, mental and physical imbalances that could take years to clear. This is why the individual needs to be patient and wait for the enlightened master.

When kundalini energy is reactivated, a person can experience a tremendous amount of heat surging throughout his body. The surging heat can be quite uncomfortable. The following remedies will cool down the internal effects of surging kundalini energy. The remedies can be applied one at a time until there is relief.

- Drink aloe vera juice.
- Mix one teaspoon of ghee (clarified butter) with one glass of warm milk and drink slowly.
- Place one tablespoon of ghee directly on the seventh chakra and gently rub it into the top of the head.
- Place ice directly on the soles of the individual's feet.
- Any or all of these remedies will slow down or stop kundalini energy from surging in the body.

Kundalini Energy and the Body

Kundalini energy created the entire universe, including the human body. It is the source of all of a person's experiences. Whatever the individual's experiences in life are, whether good or bad, happy or sad, joy or suffering, they are all the direct result of kundalini energy moving through the body. It is kundalini energy that brings the individual into this world, sustains the individual while she lives on Earth, and takes the soul away when the body dies. All of creation, on all levels, is a manifestation of kundalini energy.

Kundalini energy polarizes itself in the human body at the first and seventh chakras. Divine consciousness resides in the seventh chakra, and dense physical energy resides in the first chakra. At the seventh chakra, all the highest ideals blend into universal awareness and vibrate the truth at all times. All knowledge, bliss, awareness, peace, and joy are revealed to the individual who can hold his focus at the seventh chakra, and never let it waiver. All mental, emotional, and physical energies reside at the first chakra. This storehouse of energy directly affects the individual's entire being, including memory, ego, intellect, all past and present experiences, will-power, and all physical aspects of the body.

When the human body begins to take form in the womb, the seventh chakra is the first chakra formed by kundalini energy. Kundalini energy then moves down along the spine, creating the other main chakras. As it descends from one chakra to another, it leaves some of its divine consciousness within each chakra. The kundalini energy remains in the first chakra until it is consciously reactivated. For most individuals, the kundalini energy is not reactivated. Life goes on until death, and the individual repeats the life and death cycle over and over.

Once the kundalini energy is reactivated, it begins its upward journey back to the seventh chakra. As kundalini energy moves upward, it reconnects with the divine energy it left behind at each chakra. The chakra is then healed of any energy block or obstacle, and kundalini energy proceeds upward to the next chakra, until all the chakras are purified. When kundalini energy reaches the seventh chakra, and the individual can consciously hold kundalini energy at the seventh chakra, everything changes for the individual. Self-realization and God-realization can occur. There is complete union with the universal consciousness and the person is elevated into a state of continuous bliss. She is one with everything and no longer is separated from spirit.

If kundalini energy comes up to the seventh chakra but cannot be held there consciously, it moves downward again to one of the lower chakras. If this occurs, the person will have to clear that particular chakra before kundalini energy can move upward to the next chakra. This process is repeated until kundalini energy moves up to the seventh chakra again.

Kundalini energy is the subtlest of the subtle energies and holds the mystery of creation. It is kundalini energy that either liberates the individual or keeps him attached to the physical world. How one uses kundalini energy through his choices in life will determine what occurs for him. If a person makes choices based on fear, anger, guilt, sadness, greed, or lust, attachments to his negative energy will occur and kundalini energy will manifest negative emotional experiences. If thoughts become negative, attachments to negative thinking will occur and kundalini energy will manifest negative mental experiences. If a person becomes separated from connection to the universal energy and loses faith in spirit, attachments to negative energy will occur and kundalini energy will manifest negative spiritual experiences. Every time a person chooses to attach to a negative aspect of life, the negative energy crystallizes in that person's being. One becomes heavy, burdened, stuck. The truth cannot reveal itself so long as the veil of negativity blocks its pathway. When a person releases the negativity from his or her spiritual, mental, emotional, and physical being, a new way of life, filled with peace, harmony, joy, and happiness awaits.

Kundalini Energy and Sexual Energy

The kundalini energy system has eight main aspects: the seven chakras, and the kundalini energy itself. In the human body, kundalini energy moves upward and downward. When kundalini energy moves downward, it is often expressed as sexual energy. If the individual chooses this way of expression, a large portion of the kundalini energy will leave the body through the loss of vital fluid during ejaculation. In the *Vedas* (ancient holy books of India), it's said that it may take up to one month for the body to create vital fluid for ejaculation. If the person continues to express his kundalini energy in the downward way through sexual ejaculation, the kundalini energy can have a difficult time moving upward to the higher planes of consciousness. This will leave him with a weakened mind and body. The main goals of life will be directed toward survival and pleasures, with no energy manifesting toward union with spirit. He will not be motivated to live his life through spirit and he will live and die without ever knowing the joy and happiness of being connected to spirit.

If a person wants kundalini energy to move in an upward direction, it is essential to practice containment and control of sexual urges and activities. If one practices tantra yoga, the art of intimacy and making love without loss of vital fluids, kundalini energy will be maintained. Through the practice of tantra yoga, kundalini energy can move upward, the mind is strengthened and the body's vitality retained. People also gain increased vigor, moral fortitude, a powerful memory, and unyielding will power. Ultimately, the kundalini energy unites with the seventh chakra, and the person becomes completely liberated. Free from all worldly attachments, the person undergoes the ultimate human experience of God-realization.

Kundalini Energy and the Three Gunas

To understand the qualities of kundalini energy and how it manifests in the universal physical form, the concept of the three *gunas* was developed (guna is a Sanskrit word used to describe subtle universal energy). The three gunas are the very substances from which the physical universe emanates, and are in all things, everywhere. There is not a single physical thing in the universe that does not contain some aspect of the three gunas. Each guna has different qualities and attributes and each manifests different energies.

All three gunas manifest in the human body, however generally only one guna is dominant at any given time. The dominant guna has its own unique characteristics and qualities, and motivates the individual to make certain choices that support its particular energy. All the differences among individuals (the choices we make about life, work, play, etc.) are due to the differences in the three gunas, and how they manifest in the person. The three gunas are called *sattva guna*, *raja guna*, and *tamas guna*. Sattva, raja, and tamas are Sanskrit words meaning peaceful energy, active energy, and dense energy respectively.

When the sattva guna dominates kundalini energy within the human body, the person is at peace and experiences life in a tranquil manner. She speaks softly, walks easily, is relaxed at all times, and seeks the joy and bliss that life offers. The person is always kind, gentle, loving, and unselfish, and seeks to help humankind without any concern for reward. She is devoted to seeking and speaking the truth, and is of service to all humankind. She desires union with spirit. Acquiring worldly possessions is of no concern. Self-realization and God-realization are the end result for the person who is devoted and walks the sattvic path.

When the raja guna dominates kundalini energy within the human body, the person is active and busy. There is little time for rest and contemplation. Having the entire day planned with things to do is essential, for the person must do something to occupy his mind. His mind is agitated and there is no peace within. The restless mind creates desires for worldly things, and acquiring material possessions becomes his goal. He thinks that material things will bring him happiness, but nothing could be further from the truth. He may also be attracted to the world stage and fame and fortune. These intense desires keep him extremely busy. He might know of spiritual ideals and the concept of God-consciousness, but the attraction to the physical world is too great. He remains bound to the material world, and cannot seem to pull himself away from it. The individual's tendency is to be self-centered, thinking that the whole world revolves around him. Whatever happiness the person experiences is short-lived, because he thinks the grass is greener on the other side of the fence and he hurries on to the next thing. The concept of becoming one with spirit remains in the background of his mind, and no energy is expended in pursuit of spiritual matters.

When the tamas guna dominates kundalini energy within the human body, a person is attached to the lower, dense energies of life. She lives in ignorance and is completely attached to the inertia of life. She is stuck, inflexible, and refuses to shift her attitudes, even when the right course of action is known. She only cares about herself and will not help others. She walks, talks, and acts with great intensity. She becomes polarized in her outlook on life, making everything black or white. Rigidity in her attitudes brings rigidity to her life. The person has such dense energy that she has a difficult time understanding spiritual concepts and does not believe in love, peace, or happiness. This type of individual is uptight and refuses to change. Often, her energy is so intense that she commits crimes and does not think it is wrong to break the law.

Kundalini Energy and Karma

Karma is action in life, whether it is stored karma from a previous lifetime or present-day karma. Action is defined by how the person's physical, mental, emotional, and spiritual energies manifest into experiences and events. Whatever action an individual chooses creates karma. Actions that have beneficial effects on humankind create positive karma and actions that have detrimental effects on humankind create negative karma. All karma is stored in the chakra system. Each chakra stores karmic energy according to how the action was manifested. If the individual chooses to be self-centered, this karma will be stored in one of the lower (first, second, or third) chakras. If the individual chooses to help humankind and devotes his life in service to others, the energy of this action (karma), will be stored in one of the higher (fourth, fifth, sixth, or seventh) chakras.

When kundalini energy is reactivated and begins its upward journey, it reconnects with each chakra along the way and reactivates the energy it left behind. If the individual has any negative karma stored in any chakra when kundalini energy reactivates that chakra, it will stir the negative karma into action. The individual will then have the opportunity to clear and resolve the negative karma by learning its lesson. For example, John, who was mean-spirited to others in a previous lifetime, died without resolving his behavior through asking for forgiveness from the people he was mean to. Mean-spirited behavior was stored as negative karma in his first chakra. In this lifetime, John is sweet and kind to most people, but realizes that sometimes his behavior is rude and sarcastic, and that this behavior is unacceptable. He begins the process of changing it. He seeks professional help to resolve the deep-rooted, stuck, negative energy, so he doesn't have to act that way towards others again. John is clearing his past negative karma, and freeing the first chakra from its negative holding pattern.

Whenever kundalini energy reconnects with negative karma held at a chakra, there is an opportunity to change the karma. Often a situation that challenges the person's perspective about a certain attitude will develop, allowing the attitude to change. When attitude changes, the behavior is changed. When the behavior has changed, the negative karma is cleared.

Kundalini energy will continue to reconnect with each chakra, until all the negative karma in the entire chakra system is cleared. Enlightenment follows.

Kundalini Energy and the Nadi System

According to both yoga and Ayurvedic medicine there are about 72,000 subtle energy patterns in the body called *nadis* (nadi means movement in Sanskrit). The nadis are the vehicles of kundalini energy within the body. Without the nadi system, kundalini energy would not be able to manifest and thus the physical body would not exist. The nadis are so subtle and etheric the only way to know they exist is to feel them intuitively. When the nadis are purified, one's physical, emotional, mental, and spiritual beings are purified. This enables a person to live a more spiritual life, seeking to serve humankind and ultimately unite with spirit.

Within the nadi system, there are six main nadis that control the rest. All six nadis begin at the tip of the coccyx (tailbone), and travel up the front and back midlines of the body to the head. The three that travel up the back of the body are called *shushumna*, *pingala*, and *ida*. The shushumna nadi begins at the tip of the coccyx and travels straight up the center of the spine to the center of the top of the head. Both the pingala and ida nadis begin at the tip of the coccyx, travel upward on either side of the spine, about 1-1/2 inches from the center of the spine, to the occiput bone where the spine meets the skull. They continue traveling upward until they open into the brain, and complete their journeys at the sides of the base of the nostrils. The right-side energy nadi is the pingala, and the left-side energy nadi is the ida.

The three nadis that travel up the front of the body are called *medha*, *lakshmi*, and *saraswati* (fig 3). The medha nadi begins at the tip of the coccyx, and travels straight up the center of the front side of the body to the center of the top of the head. Both the lakshmi and saraswati nadis begin at the tip of the coccyx, and travel up the front of the body, about 1 1/2 inches on either side of the center of the body to the temporal mandibular joint where the cheek and jawbones meet at the opening of the ear. They continue to the mastoid process, the bone behind the ear, through the temporal bone to the brain and finish at the third eye. The right-side front energy nadi is the lakshmi, and the left-side front energy nadi is the saraswati. All six nadis meet at the brain center. By balancing these six nadis one balances the entire nadi system.

The pingala and ida nadis (fig. 4) are the two main nadis that carry kundalini energy through the chakra system, controlling the individual's everyday living experiences and activities. The shushumna, medha, saraswati, and lakshmi nadis remain closed and inactive during most of life. When there is spir-

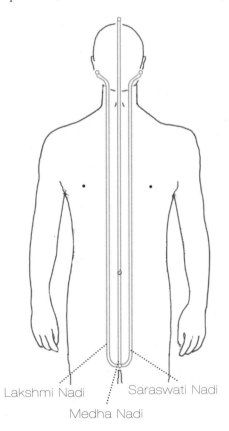

Lakshmi Nadi

Saraswati Nadi

Medha Nadi

Figure 3

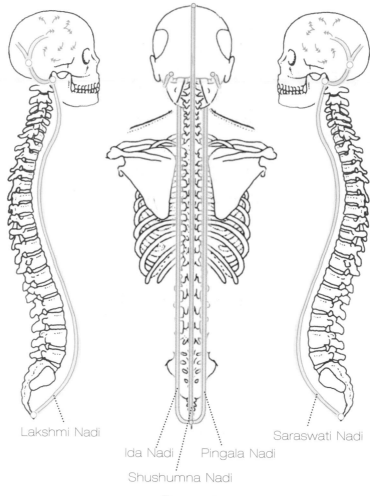

Lakshmi Nadi   Saraswati Nadi

Ida Nadi   Pingala Nadi

Shushumna Nadi

Figure 4

itual awakening in the individual, kundalini energy begins to move
through the shushumna nadi as it ascends to the seventh chakra.
Once the kundalini energy moves through the shushumna nadi, the
medha, saraswati, and lakshmi nadis become active and kundalini
energy flows through all six major nadis. As spiritual progress continues for the individual, kundalini energy operates more and more
through the shushumna and medha nadis and other nadis begin to
close down. Once the individual has progressed to self-realization,
kundalini energy is only operating through the shushumna and
medha nadis, and the other nadis completely close.

Kundalini Energy, Diet, and Climate

Kundalini energy regulates body temperature. If the body's temperature becomes too hot or cold, it can have adverse effects on how the body functions. By understanding how hot and cold foods and beverages and hot and cold climates affect the body's temperature, the individual can regulate kundalini energy.

When a person consumes cold foods and beverages, or the climate is cold, kundalini energy absorbs the cold into the body and slows the movement of kundalini energy. As a result, kundalini energy does not ascend to the head, and the mind does not receive the kundalini energy it requires. The physical body and the mind become sluggish, resulting in lethargic behavior. It becomes difficult to concentrate and the person develops an "I don't care" attitude. One has low energy and doing any kind of mental work is tedious.

When one consumes hot foods and beverages, or the climate is hot, kundalini energy absorbs the heat into the body. The heat expands the movement of kundalini energy within the body. The energy surges up into the head and the mind becomes extremely active and agitated. The overactive mind creates a state of restlessness and nervousness, resulting in the person becoming exhausted. The ability to concentrate is lost and one becomes extremely tired.

For optimum health, kundalini energy must be kept in a state of harmony and balance. Common sense, too, dictates that one wear warm clothing in a cold climate and cool clothing in a hot climate; that one not eat or drink hot, spicy foods and beverages when the weather is hot; and not to eat or drink cold foods and iced beverages when the weather is cold. When it's cold, heat-producing foods and beverages are necessary to maintain balance. When the weather is hot, cool foods and beverages are necessary.

The following breathing technique regulates cold and heat fluctuations in the body. When these fluctuations are stabilized, kundalini energy will be in harmony, and the individual will experience a state of well being.

Sit in a chair with your back straight. Inhale easily through both nostrils. With the thumb of your left hand, close off the left nostril and exhale through the right nostril. Continue to breathe through the right nostril for five full breaths. After the exhalation of the fifth breath, release your left thumb. Right nostril breathing regulates the heat of the body.

With your right thumb closing off the right nostril, repeat the technique so you are inhaling and exhaling through the left nostril. After the exhalation of the fifth breath, release your right thumb. Left nostril breathing regulates the coldness of the body.

After a while, you can increase the number of breaths to fifteen, then twenty. Practice the breathing technique three times a day for best results.

Kundalini Energy and Physical Imbalances

When kundalini energy is out of balance, the physical body is out of balance. It is kundalini energy that maintains harmony within the physical body, and any disruption to kundalini energy results in disease of the body. It is essential for optimum health that kundalini energy be free-flowing within the body. To maintain homeostasis, kundalini energy absorbs the extra heat or cold produced by the body. Kundalini energy also attaches to any threatening germ, bacteria, or virus that might attack the body and absorbs any pain that might develop. Kundalini is a self-healing energy that always seeks balance within the body. Anytime kundalini energy is disrupted, it must be brought back into balance for health to be restored.

If kundalini energy becomes cold and slows down as it travels throughout the body, many imbalances could occur. If kundalini energy becomes cold in the first chakra, the bowels may become loose and there may be pain during elimination. If kundalini energy becomes cold in the second chakra, genital nerves could be affected, making urination difficult. If kundalini energy becomes cold in the third chakra, the stomach and liver may be affected. Pain and discomfort could occur, leading to digestive disorders. If kundalini energy becomes cold in the fourth chakra, the heart and lungs may be affected. This could manifest as a form of heart disease, or feeling overwhelmed with sadness or grief. If kundalini energy becomes cold in the lungs, breathing difficulties may occur. Asthma, emphysema, or another lung disorder could manifest. If the kundalini energy becomes cold in the fifth chakra, the throat may become constricted, and the back of the neck could become tight. The ability to communicate freely could also become difficult. If kundalini energy becomes cold in the sixth chakra, the mind may become lazy and lethargic. It may not be able to focus, and concentrated mental activities could become difficult. If kundalini energy becomes cold in the seventh chakra, the ability to connect to spirit will be challenged.

If kundalini energy becomes hot it could heat up as it travels throughout the body and many imbalances could occur. If kundalini energy becomes hot in the first chakra, the nerves around the anus may become sensitive, and the veins may expand. This could result in poor circulation and hemorrhoids. If kundalini energy becomes hot in the second chakra, there may be an increased desire for sexual activity. The genitals could become overly excited, and the increased sexual activity may leave the individual exhausted. Physical stamina may be reduced, and the person may find herself weak. If kundalini energy becomes hot in the third chakra, there may be discomfort in the small intestine, resulting in constipation. Bladder and spleen difficulties could arise as well. If kundalini energy becomes hot in the fourth chakra, there may be heartburn and a rapid heartbeat. The lungs could feel as if they are burning too. If the kundalini energy becomes hot in the fifth chakra, the throat could feel dry, resulting in a constant tickle. The person may frequently clear her throat, attempting to keep it free. If kundalini energy becomes hot in the sixth chakra, the mind could become extremely active. This could lead to mental exhaustion, which could lead to physical exhaustion. One may also become burdened with worry about future events, leading to additional mental stress. If kundalini energy becomes hot in the seventh chakra, the individual will not be able to connect with spirit. When the seventh chakra becomes over-active, the individual will not be able to focus on peace, love, and happiness. Over-activity at the seventh chakra will force kundalini energy to return to a lower chakra. If this occurs, the individual would then have to clear the energy block from the lower chakra

Chapter
One:
The
Chakras

before kundalini energy has another opportunity to rise up to the seventh chakra again.

Kundalini Energy as Healing Energy

Kundalini energy is the source of everything in the universe. Not one thing exists that is not part of it. Kundalini energy enters the shushumna nadi after the individual receives spiritual initiation from the enlightened master. When the kundalini energy enters the shushumna nadi and begins its upward journey toward the seventh chakra, it connects with each chakra along the way, purifying the chakra by raising its vibrational rate and releasing any stored negative karma. No disease or imbalance can exist when the chakras are purified, and spontaneous healing can occur.

When negative karma is released from a chakra, it is called a kriya in Sanskrit. Common kriyas that might occur as the body is releasing its negative karma are yawning, laughing, crying, involuntary twitching of body parts, feeling energy movements along the spine, spontaneous rapid breathing, a feeling of hope, achieving a spiritual trance at any time of day, feeling the chakras spin, feeling heat along the spine, feeling emotional, feeling bliss, smiling, being silent, and meditating for long periods of time. When an individual experiences kriyas, it is a sign of progress and purification. Because kriyas are so unusual, the person who experiences kriyas may want to stop them from occurring. One may feel fearful, because the kriya experience is so different from anything experienced before. Do not stop the kriyas. If the kriyas are suppressed, the purification of the chakra system is suppressed, and the spiritual progress of the individual is curtailed. Kriyas usually will last about one month after spiritual initiation.

The process of reactivating kundalini energy by the enlightened master is called *shaktipat*. Shaktipat means transfer of divine energy. Of all the yogis and saints of India, only a handful of them perform shaktipat. It is a true blessing to meet such an enlightened being, and then have the courage to receive shaktipat. It is courageous to receive shaktipat because regardless of how much preparation an individual has, there is no way of knowing what one's experience will be. The shaktipat experience may be peaceful, pleasant, blissful, or trance-like, or intense, with energy surges and body movements. An individual may receive teachings from other masters, see unimaginable rainbow lights, merge with white light, or become one with all energy. It is like jumping into the water for the first time, or when a newborn baby first opens its eyes, or when an individual first experiences spirit. It is unique!

Kundalini Energy and Consciousness

The consciousness of the individual's parents at the time of his birth, the consciousness of the community, country, and world he is born into, along with the consciousness he brings from past lives, form samskaras within his chakras. These patterns determine the individual's perceptions and beliefs, and affect the choices one makes about life.

Samskara is a Sanskrit word meaning the spiritual, mental, emotional, and physical energies that follow the individual into this lifetime from past lifetimes. Yoga and Ayurvedic medicine state that up to eighty percent of all actions in this lifetime are affected by the samskaras of past lives. The remaining twenty percent is free will. What actions the individual experienced in past lives affects the individual today, in the present. What was the individual's consciousness in other lifetimes? How did he act? What were his goals? What did he accomplish? What was his purpose? Did he harm or kill anyone? Was he selfish? Did he help or serve humankind? Was he rude, angry, or sarcastic? Was he depressed? Did he have children? The list of questions goes on and on. If the person recognizes negative behavioral patterns, he may understand and conclude that he has only been acting out what he has been predisposed to do on an energy level. This might help him to understand why he is the way he is. This does not justify negative behavior toward himself or others. On the contrary, with this new awareness, perhaps the individual can program his free will to overcome his negative tendencies. The twenty percent of energy that is free will establishes a strong foundation. If the individual cultivates and harnesses his free will, he can overcome any negative tendency.

The process of clearing samskaras from the chakras can be quite challenging, since an individual has collected so many unresolved issues along the road of birth and death. The high vibrational rate of ascending kundalini energy clears each chakra from the samskaras of the past releasing a tremendous amount of energy. The samskara energy that is released could be from a positive or a negative holding pattern. If the released samskara is from a positive holding pattern, the individual will enjoy newfound energy and use it for positive things in life. If the released samskara is from a negative holding pattern, the individual will have another opportunity to clear negative energy that is holding him back from being the best person he can be. He will have to resolve the issues around the negative holding pattern, by making new and better choices in his life.

Kundalini energy does not move up to the next chakra until all the samskaras are cleared from the chakra below. If there are many issues held with samskaras at any particular chakra, the clearing process could take quite some time. It could take many lifetimes to clear the samskaras from the chakra system. However, with the grace of the enlightened master reactivating the kundalini energy, this process is usually shortened to one to five lifetimes. Once all the samskaras are cleared from the chakra system, the kundalini energy can be consciously held at the seventh chakra. The ultimate goal of enlightenment occurs for the individual who consciously holds the kundalini energy at the seventh chakra.

Kundalini Energy and Light Vibrations

The chakras continuously receive subtle light energy from the depths of the universe. Even though the individual cannot see the subtle light energy, it affects the chakra system at all times. As the chakras receive the energy, they respond either inwardly or outwardly (fig. 5). The chakras respond inwardly when their energy levels are low. The chakras use the energy to boost the overall energy level of the chakra system, bringing it back to a balanced level. The chakras can have their energy levels drained by physical, emotional, mental, and spiritual stresses, intense karma from past lives, loss of vital fluids due to overactive sexual activities, and lack of self-care. For whatever reason, it takes only one stuck chakra to create an imbalance for the rest of the chakra system.

When the chakras respond outwardly, they use the subtle light energy to help break through a negative holding pattern that is keeping the individual stuck in some destructive behavior. An energy shift occurs, resonating from the center of the body outward. A burden is lifted, and the individual suddenly feels lighter and happier. Even though it appears that nothing has really changed for the individual, her perceptions of what is going on have changed and she feels better. This often happens spontaneously. The individual's energy is transformed by a shift in how the chakra system assimilates the light energy from the universe. This light energy is always helping the chakra system achieve balance and harmony.

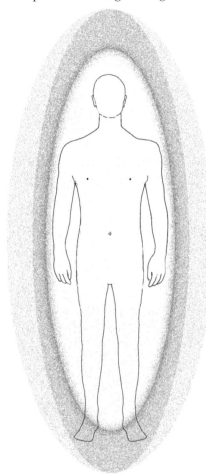

Figure 5

Chapter Two
The Chakras and You

Each chakra has a certain quality, color, sound, rate of vibration, physical, emotional, mental, and spiritual attribute. By gathering information about each chakra, a detailed picture of the human energy body unfolds. A person can then determine how the energy is manifesting through the chakra system. If the energy within the chakra system is blocked, the person will experience negative symptoms and imbalances throughout his being. If the energy within the chakra system is clear and free flowing, the person will experience happiness and peace. If an individual determines that he has energy blocks within his chakra system, he must clear these energy blocks to be happy. The process of clearing energy blocks within the chakra system takes courage, perseverance, time, energy, determination, and trust in intuition.

When an individual trusts his intuitive process, he will be able to make new choices that give him positive support. He will no longer look to others for his answers about life and he will know that he is right. He will reclaim his power and transform his life.

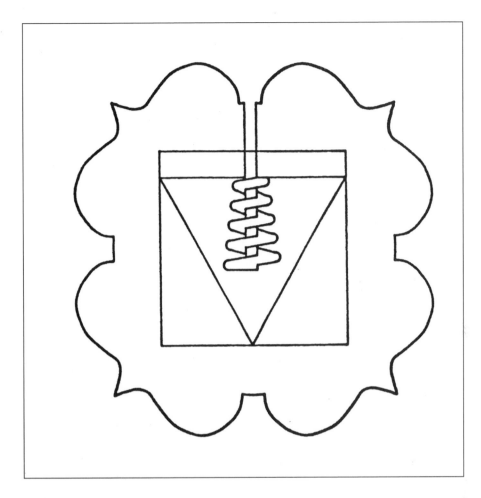

Yantra of the First Chakra

How beautiful the energy
Taking solid form.
Slow vibrations—crystallizing
Becoming whole.
Holding life together
Connected, safe, and secure.

The First Chakra

Location: At the base of the spine (the coccyx area).

Sanskrit name: Muladhara.

Element: Earth.

Sound: Lam

Sense: Smell.

Sensory organ: Nose.

Number of petals: Four.

Color: The color of this chakra is red. Red has a stimulating and invigorating effect upon the physical body. It strengthens and uplifts the internal core energy.

Body parts: Bones, especially vertebrae, teeth, hair, nails, tendons, muscles, and large intestine.

Foods: Foods that grow underground carry the Earth chakra vibration: carrots, beets, potatoes, turnips, parsnips, and radishes. (Exceptions are ginger, garlic, and onions. These foods grow underground, but due to their heating properties, they are classified under the fire chakra vibration.) White flour and white sugar products are also classified under the Earth chakra vibration because they add weight to the body.

• • •

The first chakra is the foundation of the entire chakra system. It has manifested as a dense, cohesive, solid vibratory pattern that creates the structure of the physical being. Without a strong foundation, no structure can survive for any length of time. First chakra energy is content in its density, and does not seek change or movement into another form.

First chakra energy keeps an individual grounded and attached to her roots. It represents an individual's core connection with life, and the Earth. The Earth is home; it is where an individual lives. The core of the Earth is connected to the core of the chakra system. If the Earth is in pain, people are in pain. If an individual's actions bring destruction to the Earth, she destroys herself. There is no rationale or excuse, no reward, or payoff, or monetary gain that can justify the destruction of the Earth. Anything that assists the Earth in her healing will also heal people of the Earth.

The first chakra has three zodiacal signs that correspond to its subtle energy, and each sign has a corresponding physical body part. They are Taurus the Bull, located at the throat; Virgo the Virgin, located at the large intestine; and, Capricorn the Goat, located at the knees. If the first chakra is out of balance, these three body parts might be weak and lead to various physical symptoms: constipation or diarrhea, tightness in the neck, swollen glands, or pain in the knees. There could be general muscle tightness throughout the body, pain in the bones, and a feeling of lethargy. There could also be pain in the coccyx area.

When the first chakra is in balance, there is order in a person's life. The daily routines have fallen into place, and everything in her life is organized and her living and workspace are clean and uncluttered. A wonderful flow of energy allows her to do everything she needs to do with ease. The ups and downs of life have been eliminated, and her days are filled with joyous events and experiences. She has a tremendous feeling of security and vitality, and she stays centered and secure in her identity. She is extremely healthy, and has no physical pain.

When his first chakra is balanced, a person is peaceful and remains calm during all the events and experiences of life, regardless of how they manifest. He sees life as a wonderful, enjoyable challenge and enjoys every second of every experience. He is grounded, with both feet firmly planted on the Earth and no fear of the past, present, or future. He glows with confidence, and nothing can stop him from succeeding. The Universe provides all of the individual's wants and needs and he knows this to be his truth. Everything in his life comes with ease, because he is connected to the abundance of the universal energy. There are no obstacles that are too difficult for him to overcome. The individual is happy.

When the first chakra is unbalanced with too much energy, the consciousness of the individual might be filled with illusions of grandeur. She individual might perceive herself as being irreplaceable at work, or have a tendency to dominate co-workers. She may become a workaholic, obsessed with success at all costs and never feel satisfied with what she really has. She seems to always be seeking more and more of the material world. She never quite understands that material possessions do not equal happiness.

The individual likes to work and play with intensity. He often uses drugs, alcohol, food, relationships, sex, money, and power in excess, and becomes trapped in the addictive cycle. The individual can easily jump from one addictive pattern to another. He is afraid to slow down. This leads to chaos, stress, insecurity, irritability, and confusion

This type of individual wants to control others. He tells other people where to go and what to do. This person believes the entire world revolves around him. He is a thrill seeker, and is attracted to events that produce an adrenaline high, such as sky diving, roller coaster rides, or bungee jumping. The adrenaline high covers any spiritual, mental, or emotional pain that he might be experiencing, even if the pain is subtle and he is not consciously aware of it.

When the individual recognizes that he is in spiritual, mental or emotional pain, reaching out for professional help will stop his illusion that all is well. Hopefully, his healing process will include counseling, support groups, and gentle bodywork.

When the first chakra is unbalanced by too little energy, the individual might develop rigidity, holding on to thoughts and ideas, refusing to be flexible in her belief system. This attitude can ultimately lead to a host of physical imbalances as the body tightens and contracts internally. Poor digestion, constipation or diarrhea, a weakened constitution, and low energy are the direct result of a rigid attitude. She can become so weak that she cannot perform her necessary day-to-day tasks. She loses confidence in her ability to accomplish her goals. Poor work habits could cost this person her job, and unemployment might lead to depression. She may feel unworthy of love. She may also feel unsupported, and become a loner. She may not have any interest in sex or having an intimate relationship.

A person might feel like his life is up in the air. He cannot seem to get grounded or stay centered. His mind might wander at the slightest distraction. He may become flighty and have a difficult time completing projects and meeting goals. He may worry. This worry might become so great, so emphasized that becomes burdened with the events of his own life. This attitude creates high levels of stress and is very destructive. Worry is a complete waste of energy, and it will leave a person exhausted.

The person might become inundated with fear. The fear of living and surviving in this world can be overwhelming at times. Many survival questions can arise: How am I going to live? Where am I going to work? How will my next meal manifest? If these survival questions go unanswered, the fear may intensify. When a person connects with Spirit, and trusts that all his needs will be met, fear subsides.

> I love the Earth.
> She is my home.
> She supports me
> and gives me strength
> To be.

• • •

For a complete listing of all the imbalances that are classified under the first chakra, see Appendix One; for a list of emotional imbalances, see Appendix Two.

Yantra of the Second Chakra

Abound in the ocean of joy.

Energy moving to every corner.

Satisfying, flowing freely

'Tis the water's way.

The Second Chakra

Location: Between the navel and genitals, at the sacrum.

Sanskrit name: Svadhishtan.

Element: Water.

Sound: Vam.

Sense: Taste.

Sensory organ: Tongue.

Number of petals: Six.

Color: The orange color of this chakra has a stimulating and invigorating effect upon the body. It activates the creative force and balances the passions of life. The glowing orange color recharges the desire to live life to the fullest and always be in the moment.

Body parts: Ovaries, testes, uterus, bladder, kidneys, skin, lymph glands; also the bodily fluids blood, urine, semen, sweat, tears, and cerebrospinal fluid.

Foods: Foods that grow at ground level carry the water chakra vibration: spinach, lettuce, melons, strawberries, tomatoes, cucumbers, celery, watercress, mushrooms, asparagus, chard, cauliflower, cabbage, and squash.

• • •

The second chakra is the creative center for the entire chakra system. Its vibration enhances the creative energy circulating throughout the body. It manifests as a free-flowing pattern of energy that gives the physical being pleasure.

The human body has a natural inward and outward flow of energy. The outward flow of energy begins at the central core of the chakras and vibrates outward to the aura, the electromagnetic field that surrounds the body. The inward flow of energy vibrates from the aura to the central core. Both the inward and outward flows of energy need to be in harmony for the individual to be in balance. Second chakra energy flows from the aura to the central core. Once it comes into the central core, it is distributed throughout the body. Because the second chakra corresponds to sexual energy, it is often associated with bringing the individual joy and pleasure; however, it also corresponds to creative energy, including the creative energy expressed through the arts and sciences.

The second chakra represents the connection to the waters of the Earth. Water cleanses and sustains the life of the body. Like the Earth, the human body is comprised of seventy-two percent water. If an individual's actions bring destruction to the waters of the Earth, he destroys himself. If he pollutes the waters of the Earth, he pollutes himself. There is no rationale or excuse, no reward, payoff, or monetary gain that can justify the pollution of the waters of the Earth.

The second chakra has three zodiacal signs corresponding to its subtle energy, and each sign has a corresponding physical body part. They are Cancer the Crab, located at the breasts; Scorpio the Scorpion, located at the genitals; and Pisces the Fish, located at the feet. If the second chakra is out of balance, these three body parts can be weak, resulting in various physical symptoms: lumps in the breasts, tightness in the chest, difficulties with the reproductive system like cysts on the ovaries, irregular menstrual cycles, impotency, or prostate difficulties. There can be difficulties with the feet such as fallen arches, corns, calluses, or ingrown toenails. Sometimes, there can be difficulties with the kidneys, kidney stones, urinary tract infections, or low back pain. The kidneys are one of the first organs to receive stress in the body, resulting in tired blood and eczema.

A blockage in the second chakra often results in low back discomfort or pain. Often, an individual injures her low back in what appears to be a mundane occurrence, for example, she bent over to pick up something and could not get back up, or sat in a chair the wrong way, or turned to look at something and twisted her back. At the time, these situations might seem like an accident. There are no accidents. Accidents are wonderful excuses for an individual to not accept responsibility for her actions. The truth is, at the time of the "accident" she was not paying attention to the energetic message of the second chakra. The energy of the second chakra needed to process something in some way, but she was not trained to receive such subtle messages. As a result, the second chakra manifested a

40

Balancing
the
Chakras

painful event to bring awareness there. After the person experiences pain at that chakra, she can increase her awareness at that chakra, and begin the process of healing it.

When the second chakra is in balance, a person's creativity flows joyously from one project to another with an endless supply of energy. The individual looks at the brighter side of things, and can easily find the humor in life. She laughs, plays, and is vulnerable; thoroughly enjoying herself.

The person has a carefree attitude, and regardless of what occurs, it doesn't effect him in a negative way. With such a bright outlook, he succeeds in areas that were extremely difficult for him in the past. He has tapped into the flow of life. Brainstorming new ideas and concepts is easy, and many new business opportunities appear by allowing this creative process to unfold.

The individual has a genuine sense of caring for friends and family members that allows him to really share love. This love can manifest through helping others, such as the homeless, poor, battered women, or abused children, without any regard for recognition. Relating to others in a respectful way is an easy, natural behavior. All of his feelings are easily expressed in a gentle, peaceful manner.

The person has a tremendous amount of intuitive energy, and the universe provides her with an endless supply of creative, joyous energy that she uses for the betterment of society. She has a sense of being part of the world community. One of her goals is making the world a better place to live. She takes the time to listen to her intuition and make choices accordingly. She remains in the moment and, therefore, at peace. With so much creative energy available to her, it is easy to channel it into the arts. She has a wonderful connection with spirit, and it is easy for her to receive spiritual guidance and help whenever necessary.

When the second chakra is unbalanced by too much energy, the person can be a great manipulator, and take pride in getting his way, regardless of what might happen to others. He only cares about himself and is extremely self-centered and greedy. He has the illusion that acquiring possessions and money will bring him happiness.

This attitude is ego-based and identifies only with the physical world. Whatever is acquired will never be enough. After the individual earns his first million dollars, he immediately desires his next million because he equates money with success. The only things people derive from desiring money are ignorance, unhappiness, and lack of fulfillment.

This person thinks everything and everyone around him is there for his pleasure. He believes that he is the only one who counts because he is the only one who knows what is really going on and no one else is as qualified as he. Why should he care about anyone else? Holding on intensely to this aggressive attitude wastes a lot of time and energy. It can deplete his vital storehouse of energy, making him turn to drugs for a boost.

When the second chakra is imbalanced by too little energy, the person might become afraid of people, places, and situations. The fear can block an individual's creative flow of energy, and she might become immobilized or stuck emotionally. She then becomes defensive to protect herself from the outside world. If she is constantly defensive, she keeps everyone and everything outside of her core energy. Personal relationships and intimacy become problematic and she could become a loner.

Another way a person may block his creative energy is by being overly concerned with what other people may think or feel about how him. Since no one truly knows what another person's thoughts and feelings are, it is a total waste of time to project what they might be. No one is responsible what for another chooses to think or feel. This person may deplete his energy by attempting to fix things for others, another great time-waster. Often, the person wants to fix other people because his own unresolved emotional or mental issues are triggered when listening to another's story. Rather than process his own issues, the individual focuses his attention on someone else's mental and emotional blocks, and avoids his own work by being too busy helping others.

When there is too little energy in the second chakra, the individual can become very upset at the slightest change in plans, or when he is not consulted or included in planning. He may have a tendency to go into crisis, and seems to enjoy being surrounded by drama. He has a difficult time finding motivation and may use emotional crisis for stimulation. The individual may attempt to control others by becoming the helpless victim, hoping to be rescued. The victim-rescuer cycle perpetuates crisis after crisis, because it is the only way an individual knows how to get attention. Over time, playing a victim will leave a person exhausted by the stress. The individual can also be the opposite, becoming withdrawn and shy. He does not want to attract any attention to himself, and prefers to go through life unnoticed. He chooses to hide behind his shyness, so no one will know that he is in mental or emotional pain.

> I love the water.
> She cleanses my soul.
> And connects me
> To spirit.

• • •

For a complete listing of all the imbalances that are classified under the second chakra, see Appendix One; for a list of emotional imbalances, see Appendix Two.

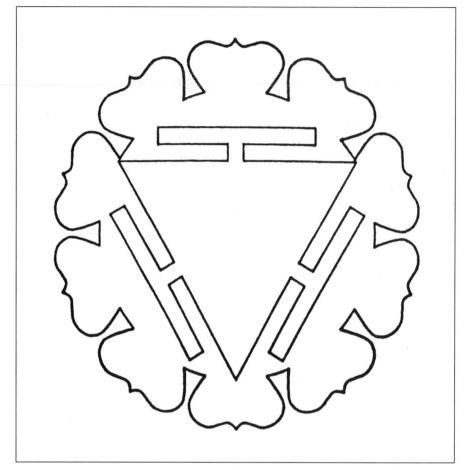

Yantra of the Third Chakra

Bursting forth with
expanding energy.
Reaching the outer depths
Of space and beyond.
Creating warmth and heat
So life can go on.

The Third Chakra

Location: At the navel center (solar plexus).

Sanskrit name: Manipura.

Element: Fire.

Sound: Ram.

Sense: Sight.

Sensory organ: Eyes.

Number of petals: Ten.

Color: The yellow color of this chakra has a warming effect upon the body. The heat that is created by the yellow color glows within the body, like the flames of a fire. It regulates digestion and controls the internal thermometer. As the flame of a candle clings to its wick so the spark of life clings to the core of being through the yellow color.

Body parts: The digestive organs, including the teeth, tongue, esophagus, stomach, liver, gall bladder, pancreas, small intestine, duodenum, and large intestine.

Foods: Foods that grow from two to five feet above the ground including rice, wheat, oats, corn, buckwheat, amaranth, quinoa, millet, barley, and rye, and hot spices including ginger, garlic, cloves, cayenne pepper, curries, and horseradish.

• • •

The third chakra creates heat for the entire chakra system. The subtle energy of the third chakra wants to expand to the outer limits of the container holding it, whether that container is the human body or the universe. As fire energy moves, it creates friction and heat. Fire energy is the source of energy for all of creation, and it is responsible for manifesting the divine energy into form. Without fire energy, nothing would exist on the physical plane. Fire energy creates the physical body, and burns the fuel of food to maintain the body. Fire energy provides an individual with the energy to accomplish all the things he desires. It travels up to the brain to give it energy to create thoughts and ideas. Without fire energy, there would not be action.

The third chakra represents our connection to the heat of the Earth. The fire energy heats the Earth, and provides warmth and nourishment to all physical bodies. The human body is no exception and cannot live without heat. If collective actions bring destruction to the heat of the Earth, we destroy ourselves. If we overheat the Earth with the accumulation of hydrocarbons or nuclear explosions, we destroy ourselves. There is no rationale or excuse, no reward, pay-off, or monetary gain that can justify the overheating of the Earth. The choice belongs to the individual!

The third chakra has three zodiacal signs corresponding to its subtle energy, and each sign has a corresponding physical body part. They are Aries the Ram, located at the head and eyes; Leo the Lion, located at the solar plexus; and Sagittarius the Archer, located at the thighs. If the third chakra is out of balance, these three body parts could be weak, resulting in various physical symptoms: cramps, gas, ulcers, colitis, heartburn, pain in the abdomen, gallstones, and liver, stomach and digestive difficulties.

When the third chakra is in balance, the expansive qualities of the fire chakra stimulate the mental capacities of thought and reason. The mind is clear of any negative thought patterns, and a person learns to make choices that serve him better. The person has direction in all his projects and clearly sees the best course of action to achieve his goals. Balanced fire energy does not allow the mind to be depressed. The individual's will power is strong and he thinks of himself as being in the flow with the universe. He believes that there is nothing that cannot be accomplished. The person is outgoing, and is always optimistic. His enthusiasm soars and he is has a cheerful nature. The individual with balanced fire energy totally believes in himself and has high self-esteem.

With a high energy level this person's capacity for right action is unlimited. A person with balanced fire energy can begin and complete as many projects as she desires. Her high energy level allows her to assume leadership roles with responsibility. She will be successful in whatever she embarks upon. Balanced fire energy allows the person to find her identity and personal power. She is relaxed, warm, friendly, and loving.

When the third chakra is imbalanced by too much energy, the individual can be overly intense about life, and need to be in control or to dominate every situation. By being dominant and telling others what to do, attention is directed to someone else, and he does not have to talk about himself, his feelings, or his personal life. He surrounds himself with a defensive wall so no one can get close and has a difficult time being vulnerable.

The individual may use her superior intelligence and highly skilled manipulation techniques to control others. She establishes an outward masquerade of superiority, dominating conversations by only talking about topics that she is familiar with. Such an individual has a huge ego, and only identifies with herself. She can be extremely demanding, and wants everyone around her to be perfect. The individual correlates the work ethic with self-worth, and strives to be the very best. She has to be number one; second place is not good enough. She does not understand why others do not have the same drive to succeed, and she perceives this lack of drive as a weakness. In her personal life, this person is very insecure and does not feel safe. She finds being vulnerable extremely frightening.

Often, the individual is very angry, and has two methods of coping with this anger: rage and silence. This is called passive-aggressive behavior, and it is an abusive behavioral pattern. The angry individual will either yell and scream, or not say a word for days or weeks at a time. His behavior is unpredictable, and it is exceedingly stressful to be around this type of individual. If the passive-aggressive person does not receive professional help, his destructive patterns will not change. Regardless of how many times he says that he will change his behavior, any positive changes will never be more than short-term.

The individual likes to make it on his own. He feels superior and resents taking orders. If pressured by authority figures, the individual may rebel. He may have difficulty holding a job. The individual is critical of others, and honestly believes that no one is as good as he. He has a difficult time admitting that he made a mistake or he was wrong. He has no compassion for those who he views as weak, and considers them to be a burden to society. He does not understand that everyone is different, and that others might not be motivated to succeed in the same way he is.

When the third chakra is imbalanced by too little energy, the person's energy level will be low because her fire energy is suppressed. She does not have the drive to fulfill her needs. She puts her goals on the back burner and has a difficult time completing projects. She may be depressed and lethargic. Sometimes she may have a difficult time getting out of bed, preferring to sleep the day away.

This type of individual feels unworthy and has little confidence in himself. He does not have strong opinions and seems to be confused. He lacks assertiveness and never gets what he wants because he never speaks up. He is very quiet, allowing others to take advantage of him. The person with too little energy in the third chakra has no healthy boundaries with which he can protect himself. Other people may come into his energy and he has no way of stopping them; he suffers the consequences. The individual does not feel like he deserves anything good in life and settles for what comes along.

A low-fire person has a tremendous fear of being alone, and rather than be alone, she will stay in an unhealthy relationship. When she is in a relationship, she has a fear of being intimate with her partner. Since she does not trust herself, it is difficult for her to trust others. Her lack of trust may foster feelings of jealousy, which can ruin any relationship.

> I love the fire.
> She warms my being.
> And gives me energy
> So I can be.

• • •

For a complete listing of all the imbalances that are classified under the third chakra, see Appendix One; for a list of emotional imbalances, see Appendix Two.

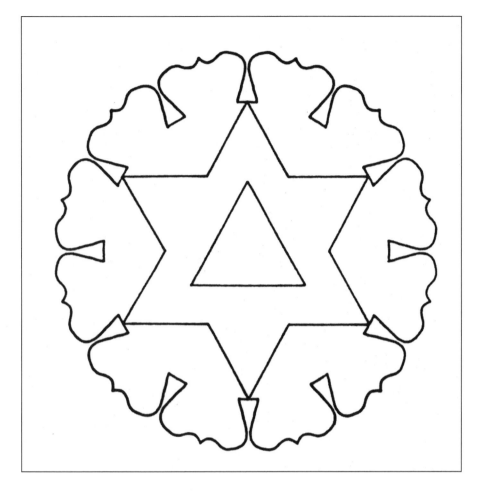

Yantra of the Fourth Chakra

From day to day
The energy circulates
Without any boundaries.
Timeless and effortless
It loves and maintains
The ongoing form.

The Fourth Chakra

Location: Chest, at the center of the sternum.

Sanskrit name: Anahata.

Element: Air.

Sound: Yam.

Sense: Touch.

Sensory organ: Skin.

Number of petals: Sixteen.

Color: The green color of this chakra has a neutralizing effect throughout the body. It regulates and soothes the etheric body, and counter-acts the effects of any negative emotions. Green is the color of the forest, which has a tranquil effect upon the soul's energy. The color green rejuvenates the respiratory and circulatory systems and has a peaceful effect throughout the physical body, balancing emotional stress.

Body parts: Heart, lungs, and thymus gland.

Foods: Foods that grow high above the ground in trees, including most fruits and nuts.

• • •

The fourth chakra represents an individual's abilities to connect to universal love energy and to feel compassion. Feeling love in a pure universal way greatly enhances the ability to connect to spirit. By feeling love, a person transcends all negativity and becomes one with all things and beings. Love is the energy that makes life worthwhile. Without love, what would life be?

Unfortunately, there are many people who remain disconnected from love and know little or nothing about it. This lack of knowledge is understandable, since the outward expression of love has been denied by generations of families in this society. In most families, it is not appropriate to ask for love, express feelings, or reach out for tenderness and receive compassion. These dysfunctional patterns of behavior have been passed down from generation to generation. There is no one to blame; it is the way it is. Born to families that lack intimacy, children learn to shut down their heart chakra, just to survive from day to day. It is almost impossible to remain open to love and be vulnerable and compassionate when living in a dysfunctional, abusive family. As an adult of the next generation, how does this child raise his children? Is he passing on these dysfunctional and abusive behavioral patterns to his children? Or can he learn to stop these inherited behavioral patterns and treat his children with love, kindness, respect, understanding, and compassion? The choice is his.

The grief of losing a loved one, the sadness of being unloved, and the hurt of losing a close relationship, can all be stored in the fourth chakra. It is not healthy to hold on to grief, sadness, and hurt for an extended period of time. The ability to love and be loved will be blocked, and there will be pain at the fourth chakra, possibly manifesting as physical heart and lung difficulties. Resolving the issues surrounding the grief, will free the energy of the fourth chakra, and allow the individual to experience love again. When the heart is healed, the joy and bliss of life return.

The fourth chakra represents an individual's connection to air energy. Air energy moves very fast and likes to jump from stimuli to stimuli. It wants to connect with new energy and have new experiences. Air energy is light, and carries the life force energy that sustains each person. No one can live without air. If our actions bring destruction to the air, we destroy ourselves. If we pollute the air with industrial wastes, we destroy ourselves. There is no rationale or excuse, no reward, or payoff, or monetary gain that can justify the polluting of the air. The choice belongs to the individual!

The fourth chakra has three zodiacal signs corresponding to its subtle energy, and each sign has a corresponding physical body part. They are Gemini the Twins, located at the shoulders; Libra the Scales, located at the kidneys; and Aquarius the Water Bearer, located at the calves and ankles. If the fourth chakra is out of balance, these three body parts can be weak, resulting in various physical symptoms: tightness at the shoulder, involving the trapezius and rhomboid muscles, scapula, and upper thoracic spine. There can also be tightness in the chest or chest pains. Any heart difficulty, including high or low blood pressure, irregular heartbeat, clogged arteries, and tightness in the diaphragm, are symptoms of a fourth chakra imbalance. Excess gas from poor digestion can travel throughout the body, lodging in muscles and bones, or creating chest pains. A block in the fourth chakra can also affect the kidneys with resulting urinary difficulties, kidney stones, low energy and fatigue. Weak ankles can cause poor posture and difficulties in an individual's gait, creating a host of structural blocks within the skeletal system, including the pelvis, low back, upper back, shoulders, neck, and head.

When the fourth chakra is in balance, universal love energy flows within a person and his heart energy reaches out to others in a compassionate, giving way. He experiences love energy on a cellular level and feels joy throughout his body. He loves himself and easily experiences his feelings. He makes self-affirming choices in life. When the fourth chakra is in balance, nothing negative enters an individual's consciousness, and his thoughts and actions remain positive. This individual has a strong desire to help others, and all of humankind, with healthy, unconditional loving energy.

Balanced heart energy results in a secure and happy individual. Others feel her heart energy and enjoy being in her presence. This individual sees the God energy in all beings and all things. She has a tremendous amount of compassion for the world, and feels connected to the plants and trees, animals, land, water, air, and people of the Earth. She is a humanitarian and sees the entire world as her home. She is enthusiastic, friendly, outgoing, and maintains a positive attitude in all situations. She has a strong sense of identity because she follows her heart energy, which helps her make healthy decisions when faced with difficult choices.

Surrendering to her heart energy is easy, and merging her love in personal relationships is natural. This individual looks forward to becoming one in body, mind, and spirit with the right partner. Her ultimate goal in relationships is merging her heart energy with her partner's spirit, and becoming one with God.

When the fourth chakra is imbalanced by too much energy, a person can be demanding, with an attitude of "wanting it all." He is never really happy with what he has, and is always looking for something else or something more, never appreciating what he already has. He cannot make up his mind and remains in limbo, or feels frustrated.

He may experience tremendous mood swings. He is either happy or sad. The constant mood swings are exhausting and can leave him emotionally weak. The individual tends to be overwhelmed with the stresses of life, not knowing how to resolve or handle difficult situations. This emotional turmoil could be stored in heart chakra.

Often, a person may put a price tag on giving love. She protects her love, guards it, sells it, but cannot seem to allow it to be. She might say, "I'll love you, if…." Her love is conditional and she uses it to control other people. Expressing love absolutely, for the sake of loving, will enable an individual to dissipate any energy block held at the heart chakra.

When the fourth chakra is imbalanced by too little energy, an individual can develop defenses and surround himself with walls that keep him from receiving love energy from others. This individual does not love himself and he does not know how to feel love. The joy in life disappears when a person becomes closed off to feelings of tenderness, openness, warmth, and happiness. Often this person is storing fear and pain from a broken heart. Deep-seated memories of feeling hurt, guilty, or ashamed linger in his heart chakra. He hides behind his fears, and lives his life mechanically going through the motions.

A person might feel lonely, because she cannot maintain close personal relationships. The possibility of being rejected stops her from taking the first step to initiate one. Often, this person assumes a victim role and feels sorry for herself when things do not go her way. It is difficult to make decisions and she vacillates from one option to another. She can feel unworthy and have very low self-esteem, a message given to her by her childhood primary caregivers. When this person develops a new set of positive values, her feelings of low self-esteem and unworthiness will disappear. The choice belongs to the individual!

I love the air.
I breathe in
Her life force energy
And it sustains me.

• • •

For a complete listing of all the imbalances that are classified under the fourth chakra, see Appendix One; for a list of emotional imbalances, see Appendix Two.

54

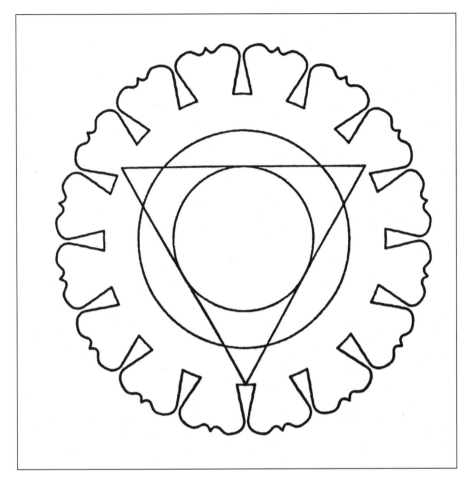

Yantra of the Fifth Chakra

Space, empty space.
To be filled
With changing forms.
Energy constantly moving
Filling the endless void.

The Fifth Chakra

Location: The throat.

Sanskrit name: Vishuddha.

Element: Ether.

Sound: Ham.

Sense: Sound.

Sensory organ: Ears.

Number of petals: Twenty.

Color: The light blue color of this chakra has a cooling effect upon the body. It is peaceful, calming, and is associated with gentleness. The light blue color will soothe the neck and throat. It can assist in helping people speak the truth.

Body parts: Throat; thyroid and parathyroid glands.

Foods: This is a very high vibrational energy center, and does not really have many foods associated with it. Foods that carry this vibration are limited to blueberries, purple cabbage, and plums.

• • •

The fifth chakra creates space for the manifestation of all the physical elements. The fifth chakra is the master chakra. When the human body determines that it needs more of one element or less of another to maintain its homeostasis, the elements shift from one to another via the fifth chakra. The fifth chakra is the neutral zone, it provides the energy space in which elements transmute. All elemental changes that are required by the body occur through the ether chakra.

The mind controls the ether chakra, and the ether chakra controls the physical body. That is why the ether chakra is said to be the bridge between the higher, spiritual sixth and seventh chakras, and the lower, physical chakras. The ability to communicate is centered at the ether chakra, where speech originates. If an individual has difficulty expressing the desires and needs of her lower physical chakras, the ether chakra will be effected.

The fifth chakra represents the connection to the space of the Earth. Without the container of space to hold energy, the Earth would not exist. Space makes Earth the vehicle that manifests the other elements of, earth, water, fire, and air into physical form. If an individual's actions bring destruction to the space of the Earth, the planet will not survive. There is no rationale or excuse, no reward, payoff, or monetary gain that can justify the destruction of the space of the Earth.

The fifth chakra is vibrating at such a fast pace, it moves beyond the physical representation of the Zodiac. The fifth chakra correlates to the space of the body, which is less tangible than the physical elements of the zodiac. The fifth chakra energy can be difficult to grasp because it is so subtle. It is like attempting to wear the wind. One can feel the wind, but it is impossible to hold on to it. The fifth chakra does correlate to the throat and thyroid and parathyroid glands, and the body spaces that hold these organs. The fifth chakra is often visualized as a triangle, and on a structural level, the skeletal system finds its balance through the occiput, sacrum, and heel bones, which are the three main triangular shaped bones of the body. They give the body strength and balance when they are in alignment with one another and give the skeletal system the space it needs to function.

When the fifth chakra is in balance, living in the moment is simple and effortless. Day-to-day decisions concerning self-care and gentle living come easily. The lower chakras function clearly, and the individual can focus his attention toward connecting with spirit. The individual is in the right place at the right time; success comes easily.

This individual's ability to communicate is enhanced, and other people listen to what he has to say. The individual experiences great joy learning to commune with spirit. The person only speaks the truth, and his spiritual knowledge is used for the betterment of society. When a person is honest and remains loyal to his convictions, harmony prevails.

Maintaining a conscious awareness of the fifth chakra offers a person new opportunities to become free from old negative conditionings. As an individual becomes aware of her old negative patterns, she begins to make healthier choices that effect her life in a positive way. The individual learns from past mistakes, and frees herself from deep-rooted uncertainty, self-doubt, and low self-esteem.

When the fifth chakra is in balance, life is wonderful. The individual is centered, knows what he wants out of life, and can achieve his goals with ease. Communication with others is effortless, and he can articulate his deepest spiritual knowledge to others. This individual learns how to use spiritual energy in prayer and devotional ceremonies to achieve high states of meditation. The individual quickly grasps spiritual concepts and ideas, and applies these spiritual teachings in his life. He is in control of his energy and does not waste it on feeling negative emotions or thinking negative thoughts.

When the fifth chakra is imbalanced by too much energy, the individual talks endlessly about many unrelated subjects. He talks for the sake of talking, not realizing how much energy he is wasting. He may have intense conversations about politics, religion, current events, or sports that just seem to go round and round without any purpose, never resolving anything.

Constant communication about the small details of every experience in life keep this person so occupied he can never really communicate his feelings. A person's feelings help determine who he is and it is vital for an individual's emotional well being to communicate what he is feeling.

Sometimes, this person wants to impress others with her knowledge of specific subjects. She has a strong need for approval and ego-strokes. She prefers to be around people she can dominate and control with his wit or knowledge.

When the fifth chakra is imbalanced by too little energy, the individual is passive, quiet, timid, shy, and does not want to be in situations where she has to express anything about herself. The individual is inconsistent in action, without the motivation to follow through. This person is exhausted quickly. The individual is petrified to reveal herself, and holds back at work, sex, and in relationships. This individual settles for second best, never realizing her potential. She is the perpetual wallflower, scared to step forward and remaining in the background. This person is nervous and uptight in most situations that involve other people.

This type of person could lose his identity, self-respect, and self-worth and fall into a depression. Depression may drastically alter the person's ability to function in a holistic way. He retreats behind a lethargic "whatever" attitude and loses the ability to care for himself. If the depression goes untreated he may eventually lose his desire to live.

Because this person does not have the tools to express himself, he sometimes attempts to manipulate other people. He might tell five different stories to five different people about the same topic. When they compare stories no one knows what is really going on. If anyone confronts him about his behavior, he will act confused, make up excuses, or get defensive to cover himself. By confusing others, he is the only one who really knows what's going on. He then feels in control and safe. When he feels safe, he does not have to feel his feelings of emotional or mental pain.

> I love space.
> It gives me form
> So I can change
> And become one
> With the universe.

• • •

For a complete listing of all the imbalances that are classified under the fifth chakra, see Appendix One; for a list of emotional imbalances, see Appendix Two.

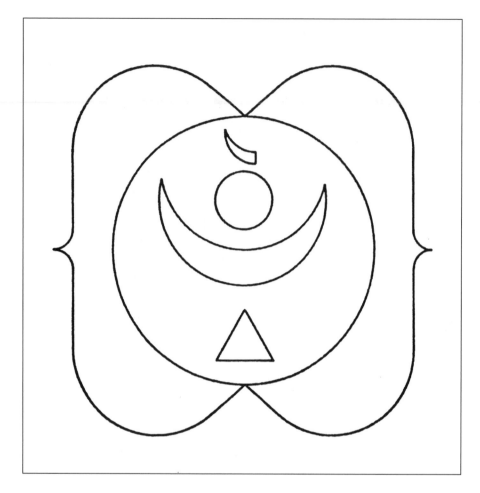

Yantra of the Sixth Chakra

How incredible
To see the universe
With eyes closed.
To know all knowledge
And feel every feeling.
To be one with your soul.

The Sixth Chakra

Location: In the middle of the forehead.

Sanskrit name: Ajna.

Sanskrit name: Light.

Sound: Om.

Sense: Thinking.

Sensory organ: Mind.

Number of petals: Two.

Color: The deep blue indigo color of this chakra activates the individual's intuitive powers and increases his mental clarity and his psychic capabilities. The indigo color has a cooling effect upon the physical body and helps purify the blood. The indigo color can assist the healing of many mental disorders, especially obsessions.

Body parts: The pituitary gland, brain, eyes, and ears. The sixth chakra is a very high vibrational energy center and the number of physical aspects associated with it are limited.

Foods: The sixth chakra is the mental energy center and does not have any foods associated with it.

• • •

The sixth chakra is often called "the mind's eye" because it controls the perception and assimilation of light and color. The sixth chakra vibrates at such a high degree that it transcends the quality of time. The individual who has gained mastery of the sixth chakra can energetically travel into the past and future in order to access information from past lives and obtain new awareness about the present. Everyone is born with karma from other lives. This new awareness helps a person understand present day energy blocks throughout her chakra system and resolve the underlying issues in a gentle way. Once the blocks are resolved, she can experience universal truth and her soul will be set free.

Sixth chakra energy is beyond the physical dimensions of the five lower chakras. The easiest way to get in touch with sixth chakra energy is through the intuitive process. Once the individual's intuition is activated, she will be able to see the human aura as different colors, which represent different energies and qualities of the body. By observing the rainbow colors of the aura, the individual can locate the indigo of the sixth chakra.

The sixth chakra is commonly called the *ajna* chakra. *Ajna* is a Sanskrit word meaning, to have command or control of. When applied to a human's potential, it means to have control of his thought processes. A person's perception of life clears as her psychic pathway opens, bringing freedom to her mind. When the mind is free of unwanted, negative mental energy, the truth reveals itself effortlessly, as the sixth chakra energy opens and blossoms like a rose.

Thoughts are energy, a person with clarity and knowledge of his thoughts can use their energy to control the slower-moving energy of his lower chakras. A person is what he thinks. By controlling his mental thoughts, he is able to create thought patterns that are healthy and positive. By avoiding negative thought patterns, he can avoid negative actions.

The sixth chakra represents the individual's connection to the creative energy that manifests through his intuition, psychic pathways, clairvoyance, and mental clarity. Without intuition, a person has difficulty making healthy choices. Without the use of his psychic and clairvoyant ability, he does not know about his past or future. If the individual misuses his sixth chakra energy for personal gain, he slows his spiritual growth. There is no rationale or excuse, no reward, or payoff, or monetary gain that can justify an individual's conscious blocking of spiritual energy. The choice belongs to the individual!

When the sixth chakra is not in harmony, the pituitary gland, eyes, nose, and ears are affected. The pituitary is the master gland and regulates all other glands. Any imbalance to the pituitary gland may lead to a yin/yang effect upon the body's energy, swinging it from high to low energy. Other problems that can occur are difficulties with hearing, seeing, and mental clarity.

Balanced sixth chakra energy allows an individual to find life's rhythm and easily go with the flow. He lives in harmony with his environment, and is deeply connected to nature. He relies on spirit to guide him, and meditates. He sees all things with his eyes closed, he knows without asking questions, feels without touching, and listens without hearing. He has the ability to become one with cosmic consciousness and receive universal love energy. This person is a leader, and guides others by living a life of integrity. He is not attached to the results of his actions and prays to spirit before engaging in any activity. He lives through his spiritual energy, receiving internal bliss from his direct contact with the universal love energy. His connection to spirit remains unswayed by worldly distraction. All knowledge of the universe is available to him, and he sees the past, present, and future simultaneously.

This person has mastered the skill of meditation and can leave his body to become one with the universal energy in the depths of space. The ability to consciously leave the body in meditation resolves the fear of death, which is understood as the transition from one manifestation of divine energy to another. This person is at peace with the knowledge that the soul is eternal, and it is only the physical body that comes and goes in death and rebirth. When the individual's Earthly karma is resolved, and all his lessons of life have been learned, the individual no longer reincarnates into another physical body. The soul then manifests its form on the astral plane. When its astral karma is complete, the soul next manifests its form on the causal plane. When the causal karma is complete, the soul permanently merges with the universal consciousness and becomes one with all.

When the sixth chakra is imbalanced by too much energy, the individual identifies with ego and a pervasive sense of me. He believes no one can do better than he can and he resents all those who try. He is not in touch with the truth, and makes choices based on his illusions. He is living in the world of *maya*, the Sanskrit word for illusion. Most people live in maya, unconnected to spirit, and identified only through the body and the physical world.

This person identifies with his ego so strongly he must be right about everything. He will argue each and every point of a conversation until he wins. His life is a power struggle and he may bring law-suits to prove that he is right. Nothing is his fault and he blames others for his unhappiness. Anyone who gets in his way will be abused and he will feel no remorse.

When the sixth chakra is imbalanced by too little energy, the individual does not have the discipline to complete projects, and becomes fragmented in her work. She is fearful about success, getting what she wants, and about being alone. It is difficult for her to talk about her fears and she remains quiet. She chooses to live through other people's feelings. She may seems sensitive, but is actually in denial of her own feelings. It feels much safer not to own her feelings.

She fears being hurt and has a difficult time trusting other people. She lacks direction and appears as if she is half-asleep. She lacks enthusiasm, does not have a high regard for herself and sees herself as unworthy. Nothing positive happens to her. She cannot take charge of any situation, even if her life depends on it. She prefers to be passive and helpless, liking the victim role.

> I love the third eye.
> She gives me knowledge
> Of the past, present, and future.
> She allows me to see, and know
> Everything.

• • •

For a complete listing of all the imbalances that are classified under the sixth chakra, see Appendix One; for a list of emotional imbalances, see Appendix Two.

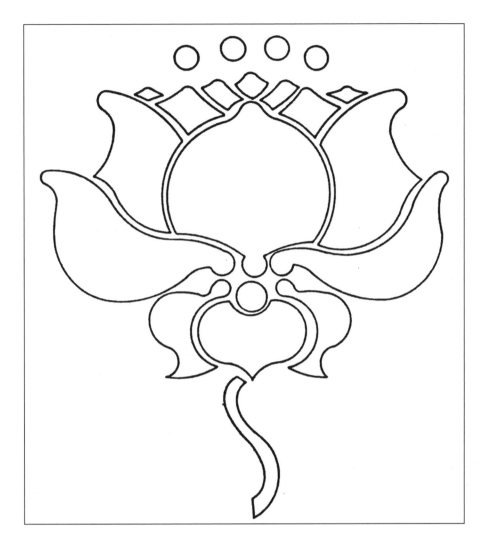

Yantra of the Seventh Chakra

The past, the present, the future.

Is there any difference.

Everything is one.

The ultimate joy

Merging all energies

With the supreme consciousness.

Merging completely with God.

The Seventh Chakra

Location: The top of the head.

Sanskrit name: Sahasrara.

Element: Super-Consciousness.

Sound: Aum.

Sense: Spirit.

Sensory organ: Brain.

Number of petals: One thousand.

Color: The violet color of this chakra has a soothing effect upon the nervous system. Violet is calming and helps the body relax deeply. People suffering from depression receive a tremendous healing from this color. Violet represents the individual's connection to spirit, and assists in feeling peace, wholeness and tranquillity.

Body parts: The pineal gland and the brain.

Foods: Meditation is the real food of life. The seventh chakra represents the spiritual energy of the body. Its vibration is moving so fast, it is beyond association with food. This chakra nourishes the body through meditation and unification with spirit.

• • •

The seventh chakra is the master of the chakra system, responsible for the well being of the individual's physical body and spiritual soul. It represents the pure universal consciousness that resides within the body. The vibration of the seventh chakra is moving so fast it manifests as pure spirit. The seventh chakra has been described as the seat of super-consciousness. All emotions, physical elements, thoughts, and vibrations merge with the universal energy into one form. Within the seventh chakra, there is no separation, classification, or categorization of energy; all is one.

The energy of the seventh chakra represents the individual's cosmic link to the universal consciousness. It is so subtle that the only way to become aware of its energy is to cultivate the qualities of love, hope, charity, peace, joy, and inspiration.

Awareness of the seventh chakra brings freedom to the soul. The seventh chakra's energy is not limited by the physical laws of nature.

It operates by the spiritual laws of the universe—cultivating love, compassion, faith, hope, inspiration, aspiration, intuition, truth, and all-knowledge. When a person lives life through spiritual laws, a complete state of union with all things and a continuous feeling of bliss are achieved. All karma is resolved, and she can consciously leave the physical body, and merge with spirit any time she desires.

Without the seventh chakra's connection to the universal cosmic energy, a person would be lost. Without the guidance of the universal cosmic energy what would a person do? What direction could a person go? How could she survive? If her actions disconnect her from the universal cosmic energy, she destroys herself. There is no rationale or excuse, no reward, payoff, or monetary gain that can justify an individual's disconnection from the universal cosmic energy. The choice belongs to the individual!

The seventh chakra governs the pineal gland, which assimilates light vibrations from the universe and directs them into the body. When the pineal gland is out of balance, an individual may have a lack of enthusiasm, loss of confidence and vitality, and low energy. The person may become sickly.

When the seventh chakra is in balance, universal love energy easily vibrates into the individual. The person lives through the higher spiritual laws of love, peace, hope, and charity. She only speaks the truth and inspires humankind to live up to its highest potential. Her entire being is uplifted, and the lower chakra energies of attachments, desires, greed, and lust are eliminated. In the presence of such a being, an individual is filled with love energy, and his worldly difficulties or problems disappear from his consciousness. What a blessing to be completely filled with universal love energy in every cell, muscle, organ, and bone.

The higher spiritual vibrations of the seventh chakra manifest energy in an etheric light form so subtle it is impossible to hold, shape, or mold it on the physical plane. The only way to access this type of energy is through meditation when the mind is quieted and concentration is enhanced. The cosmic consciousness of the universe is then experienced directly throughout the entire physical body. This is extremely healing. All of life's questions are answered, and joy is experienced at the highest level possible.

When the seventh chakra is imbalanced by too much energy, the individual may feel like he is lost in society, and does not fit in with any group of people. He does not relate well or understand why people do not like him. Tremendous frustration can ensue, leading to depression, migraine headaches, or lethargy. He may be sarcastic or rude. He person might feel like he is always missing something, or just out of sync. This person is not connected to spirit, and is closed off from happiness, other relationships, dreams, reality, truth, and from his connection to the universal love energy.

When the seventh chakra is imbalanced by too little energy, the individual takes life too seriously and stops having fun. There is no joy in life—it is filled with burdens. The individual might slouch under the weight of constant worry and unresolved stress, or may be slovenly and stop eating properly. Her poor diet leads to even lower energy and lethargy. She likes to escape into her own world where she does not have to relate to others. She builds a wall around herself.

> I love the cosmic consciousness.
> She gives me freedom
> To be with everything
> Forever and forever.

For a complete listing of all the imbalances that are classified under the seventh chakra, see Appendix One; for a list of emotional imbalances, see Appendix Two.

68

Balancing
the
Chakras

Chapter Three
Healing and Transformation

The Universal Law of Conscious Thought

Every thought an individual thinks or speaks sends a vibration throughout the universe that eventually returns to the sender. By cultivating negative thoughts, a person manifests negative experiences. By cultivating positive thoughts, a person manifests positive experiences.

A person's mental intentions are vital to becoming one with spirit. A person must learn to be united in spirit and center all of his thoughts and actions in spirit. He will then be able to manifest the perfection of spirit in everything he does and says. However, if he is absorbed in his ego and the physical world he will manifest attachment, burden and suffering. When the individual is ready to comprehend that everything of this world is spirit, he will see spirit in all things.

Life's Rhythm

The rhythm of the universe is everywhere, in everything. It originates in the depths of space and moves throughout the universe, expanding and contracting. Its constant movement creates a pulse that permeates all aspects of creation. Every manifestation of energy is ruled by the universal rhythm.

In the human body, the universal rhythm expands from its central core to the aura, and from the aura back to the central core. If an individual closes his eyes and becomes quiet, he can feel the universal rhythm within his body. Once he connects with the internal pulse he can begin to change his vibrational essence. With conscious internal movement of the universal rhythm he can release negative holding patterns. This enables his cells to transform their energies and free themselves of any imbalances or diseases that might have been developing within their structures.

If you have any difficulty in finding the universal rhythm within yourself, pay attention to your breath when your body is relaxed. The rhythm of the breath is identical to the universal rhythm. As you observe your breath, you can feel the rhythm of your body. Being connected to the universal rhythm will connect you to spirit. You will feel one with the universe.

Rejoicing the Transformation

At last, the time has come for some individuals to begin their transformation into the light and behold the cosmic universal consciousness. It is a joyous time when the evolution of the soul begins to shine brightly with the light; a light that is one with all of creation. It is a time to release doubts, fears, anger, frustrations, and desires that block the light from shining within and without.

When a person holds firm in her thoughts that all in creation is spirit, there is no separation from the cosmic light. Until that realization totally permeates every action and thought, she will remain separated from spirit. In that separation, she will long to be loved, to be fulfilled, to be at peace, to be in harmony, to be happy, and to be blissful. In that separation, she collects things, thinking that happiness is found by possessing material goods. She indulges physical desires, thinking that happiness is found in physical satisfaction. She seeks comfort in others, not realizing that only her connection to spirit can soothe her soul.

To behold the cosmic light, remember, all thoughts come from the cosmic light. All things are a manifestation of thoughts. Send your lower thoughts of pride, lust, jealousy, anger, shame, greed, and unworthiness back to the cosmic light. Be relentless with your determination, and repeat the process for every negative thought, until the negative thoughts no longer arise in the mind. Concentrate, and hold firmly the thoughts of harmony, love, and bliss. Happiness will follow!

Chapter
Three:
Healing
and
Trans-
formation

The Healing Process

The journey of self-healing is an enriching road to travel upon. Often, a life-threatening situation propels an individual into the healing process. The individual might suddenly discover that he has manifested a serious physical or emotional imbalance. Statements like, "My life has become unmanageable," or "I can't take the pain anymore," indicate that the individual is ready to heal himself.

Healing requires a tremendous effort. It takes commitment, clarity, perseverance, and determination. Ayurvedic medicine states that for every year of imbalance, it takes one month of conscious effort to heal that imbalance. The healing journey often takes some time because the individual may have been out of balance longer than he realizes.

The Healing Crisis

A healing crisis occurs when the body, mind, and spirit of an individual come into balance from a point of imbalance. The individual's soul current carries the memory of all events experienced during this lifetime and past lifetimes, and stores it in the individual's chakras and the cells of the body.

When the individual begins to heal herself, whether through bodywork, affirmations, emotional stress release, counseling, or, meditation, the stored energetic memory of her negative life experiences are released back into the blood stream for purification. When the stored negative energy is released into the blood stream, the body can have a slight setback and not feel well. This is the healing crisis. The body reacts to this flood of toxins being suddenly released into the system by filtering the toxins through the liver, kidneys, lymph system, and skin. It usually takes from two to eight hours for the body to filter through most of the toxins. As this purification occurs, the individual might experience temporary symptoms of illness such as headaches, upset stomach, slight fever, anger, sadness, or crying. It is not cause for worry. The symptoms pass and the person feels much better in a short period of time.

Rest helps. It is very important to drink as much water as possible when the healing crisis first occurs, as it will help flush the toxins from the tissues and keep the internal healing energy moving so it can continue to eliminate all of the released toxins.

Clearing Emotional Imbalances

An individual is comprised of spiritual, mental, emotional, and physical energies that interact at all times. It is impossible to separate one from the other. What occurs for one aspect of an individual's being affects all. An individual may be unaware of the stresses to his spiritual, mental, and emotional beings. Internal stress can be very difficult to recognize, but the physical body responds to these stresses by manifesting physical symptoms or diseases. The sequence does not change: the physical body does not develop a disease or ailment without having unresolved spiritual, mental, and emotional stresses preceding it.

When a person takes a deep look inside and recognizes that he is comprised of these many different aspects, he can begin to balance them as he seeks wholeness. If the individual is in denial and refuses to acknowledge that he is comprised of spiritual, mental, emotional, and physical energies, he may manifest pain and suffering without ever knowing why. It will be difficult to heal because he will not know where to begin or how to proceed. Each time an individual manifests a physical symptom, it is up to him to realize that there is unresolved stress that caused the pain or symptom to manifest on the physical level. A person has to understand this concept and take the necessary actions to clear his imbalances. The choice belongs to the individual.

A person can reconnect to spirit and heal his spiritual being through pranayama, chanting mantras, and meditation. He can heal his mental being of all negative thoughts by using positive, angelic affirmations and understanding his personality tendencies through astrology, and heal the physical being by using homeopathy, herbal teas and tinctures, yoga asanas, aromatherapy, mudras, and diet. There are four steps that enable an individual to come into harmony from emotional imbalances:

73

Chapter
Three:
Healing
and
Trans-
formation

1. Identify the feelings from any unresolved emotional stress.
2. Feel the feelings.
3. Grieve the loss of the relationships that could have been.
4. Forgive yourself and others from your heart.

1. Identify the feelings from any unresolved emotional stress.
An individual has to be able to identify his feelings before he can come into balance with them. This can be extremely difficult because people do not know how. In most families of origin, feelings were not discussed or expressed. There was no healthy and appropriate way for children to express their feelings because their primary care-givers, usually their parents, did not know how to do it themselves.

Most caregivers were concerned with feeding, clothing, and pro-viding shelter for their children. Who had time for feelings when life was about satisfying basic survival needs? Their parents, who learned it from their parents, passed down this attitude to them. Our ancestors had to endure great hardships on the physical plane and as a result their priorities shifted into concerns of physical sur-vival. Emotional concerns and happiness were not a priority. These attitudes have been passed on to subsequent generations. As a result, many contemporary families do not know how to express their feel-ings in a healthy way.

When someone in a family begins to receive professional help, the dysfunctional emotional behavioral patterns start shifting. One family member can help other family members get help too. It may be a slow process, involving many generations of family members, before the entire family is relating to feelings in a healthy way.
In this process of emotional clearing there are eleven feelings that will be identified: anger, hurt, sadness, loneliness, guilt, fear, shamed, joy, bliss, peace, and happiness.

A simple exercise will assist an individual with identifying his feelings at any given moment. It will also give the individual insight to his emotional being:

At five different times throughout the day, stop what you are doing, sit in a chair, close your eyes, and ask yourself, "How do I feel?" Write down the particular feeling or feelings that you feel at that moment (use the above mentioned eleven feelings as a guideline). Do not be attached to any of the feelings that are recorded. Continue this process for two weeks. At the end of the two weeks, you will be able to identify your feelings at any given moment.

2. Feel the feelings.

An individual may stop feeling emotions early in childhood. Her primary caregivers might have responded to her emotional expressions in an abusive manner. She may have been belittled, put down, yelled at, beat up, made fun of, ridiculed, or her parents might have responded with guilt, shame, or anger. She learned to survive her childhood by suppressing her feelings and emotions. It was her choice.

As an adult, this individual lacks the confidence to express her feelings because she is still stuck in her childhood pattern. This is sad, but it is the truth. When she rediscovers her feelings, she will recapture his emotional identity and being.

As the individual begins to feel, she becomes vulnerable. This vulnerability brings her strength of character and the ability to make self-supporting choices. This is the opposite of what people usually think: that if an individual is vulnerable, she is weak and will be taken advantage of. This is not true. By staying in touch with her feelings the individual will have the dignity and grace to be in balance emotionally and achieve emotional clarity.

3. Grieve the loss of the relationships that could have been.

People do not feel safe around family members, co-workers, or friends who exhibit dysfunctional behavioral patterns. As a result they stop communicating their feelings and create distance in these relationships. Intimacy is lost and these relationships can not develop in closeness, love, or peace. As a result, people drift away. Family members or friends move away to avoid contact and sometimes choose not talk to one another at all because the pain is so deep. A person needs to grieve the loss of these close personal relationships. By grieving the loss of these relationships, the blocked energy can be transformed.

Most people do not realize how much emotional energy it takes to hold on to the pain of these old, dysfunctional relationships. Only after the individual lets go does she realize the enormous amount of energy it took to maintain her attachment to them. If the individual can free herself of attachments to old relationships, she can set her soul free.

4. Forgive from the heart.

When an individual forgives from his heart, he completes the process of healing his emotional being. Forgiving from the heart means that the individual is willing to let go of the remaining negative emotions from his past dysfunctional relationships. He is then ready to make amends with his friends and family members, and move on with his life in a positive manner.

For this process to really work, it is necessary to complete all four steps. If an individual only completes one or two of the steps, he will not complete his journey and will probably find himself facing the same issues again in the future. (A list of the negative emotional qualities of the chakras can be found in Appendix Three.)

Setting Healthy Boundaries

Setting a healthy boundary is the next step in healing. Setting a healthy boundary is a way that an individual can say, "Stop, that behavior hurts." The main goal of setting a boundary is to stop one individual from imposing negative, intense, unwanted, dysfunctional behavior upon another. The individual who sets the boundary needs to accomplish this in a gentle, loving way. He wants to consciously respond to the unwanted behavior, instead of mindlessly reacting to it. The following steps help the individual accomplish his goal.

1. Use "When you do that, I feel this." statements.
2. Be clear about what behavior is acceptable and what is not.
3. State the boundary clearly.
4. Follow though on the boundary.

1. Use "When you do that, I feel this." statements.

By using the, "when you do that, I feel this" technique, an individual can calmly state his feelings about any unwanted behavior from another person. This technique is simple and easy to do. The only prerequisite is that the individual be able to identify his feelings clearly. Once a person knows what he is feeling, he can easily say, "stop, that hurts," or "I feel scared, please do not do that again."

2. Be clear about what behavior is acceptable and what is not.
Unacceptable behavioral is that which is hurtful and abusive:

Physical abuse is *anything* done to your body without your consent. Any invasion of your physical boundaries or your body constitutes physical abuse.

Sexual abuse is any sexual invasion of either your physical or emotional boundaries without your consent. This ranges from the overt rape, to the covert sexual innuendo, or deprivation of privacy.

Emotional abuse is a violation of your emotional boundaries. Violent language, sarcasm, destructive criticism, silence, and neglect all constitute emotional abuse. Whenever your own unique emotional reality is denied or discounted, you are being emotionally abused.

Intellectual abuse occurs when your opinions and ideas are ignored, discounted, or ridiculed. You have the innate right to think for yourself, formulate your own opinions, puzzle things out, and make mistakes. When your intellectual processes are interrupted or interfered with, that is intellectual abuse.

Spiritual abuse is a bit trickier to define because it usually involves one or more of the above. Every individual has a need for and a right to love, attention, direction, affection, and support. They are necessary to spiritual development. Whenever an individual's boundaries, physical, sexual, emotional, or intellectual have been violated, he has been spiritually abused as well.

3. State the boundary clearly.
The person states the boundary he is going to use to protect himself from the unwanted behavior. This usually means getting away from the person who is displaying abusive behavior.

4. Follow though on the boundary.
If the unwanted behavior does not change, the individual follows through with his boundary.

77

Chapter
Three:
Healing
and
Trans-
formation

. . .

For example, Joe is a drinker. When Joe drinks, he becomes rude, sarcastic, and yells at his wife Mary. He has promised Mary that he will not drink anymore. Joe realizes that his drinking has affected his relationship with his wife in a negative way (no one wants to be around someone who is drunk), and he is attempting to stop his drinking. But Joe is not seeking professional help and is attempting to change his behavior with strong determination. One month later, Joe comes home with alcohol on his breath. Mary confronts him about his drinking and Joe apologizes. Mary then sets the following boundary: "Joe, when you came home tonight with alcohol on your breath, I felt hurt, sad, and ashamed. As a result of your unacceptable behavior, I am going to take care of myself by going to an Alanon meeting." (Alanon is a support group for family and friends of alcoholics.) As a result of his behavior, Joe knows his wife's feelings were hurt. She did not want to be around him and needed to go to a support group for help. He knows he has to stop drinking or risk the chance of alienating his wife again.

Mary responded in a healthy way. She calmly expressed her feelings about Joe's negative behavior and stated what she was going to do to take care of herself. If Joe continues to drink, Mary will have to continue to set tougher and tougher boundaries. Mary's next boundary might be stating how she feels about his drinking, then telling him that she is going to Alanon, and then leaving the house for half a day. Mary's next boundary might be going to a counseling session and leaving the house for the whole day. With each episode of Joe's dysfunctional, unwanted behavior, Mary will spend more and more time away from him. If Joe's drinking does not stop, Mary will probably have to leave permanently. If Mary does leave the relationship, it will be the correct decision. Ultimately, Mary has to take care of herself, and get away from the abusive situation with her husband. No one deserves to be abused.

If a person finds herself in an abusive situation, she must attempt to stop the abuse. If she can not stop the abuse, she must leave the abusive situation. No one needs to be around people who choose to abuse them. The choice belongs to the individual.

79

Chapter
Three:
Healing
and
Trans-
formation

Chapter Four
Self Help for the Chakras

This self-help section is designed to assist an individual in healing her chakra system. There are many holistic ways to bring the chakra system into balance and one way of healing isn't better than another way. An individual chooses the method of healing to suit her needs. Healing is a journey. It is important to go slow and easy. There is no set time for healing. Ayurvedic medicine states that it will take one month of conscious effort to heal each year of imbalance. When embarking upon the healing journey, avoid being in process all day long, it will leave a person completely exhausted. If a person becomes tired, resting for a while is recommended. The person can then restart the process at a more manageable pace.

Throughout this section, I give examples of various techniques. As I describe the modalities I use the word, "practitioner." As I use this word, I am referring to the person who is doing the healing technique, and not necessarily to a trained professional.

Polarity Balancing Body Work

Gentle polarity-balancing bodywork is a wonderful way to heal the chakra system. It can release past karma, relax all of the body's different energy systems, and facilitate a true sense of well being in the individual. In the polarity balancing healing system there are basic energy principles that underlie the electrical dynamics of the body. The upper part of the body—chest and higher—has a positive electrical charge. The middle part of the body—thighs, hips, and belly—has a neutral electrical charge. The lower part of the body—knees and lower—has a negative electrical charge. Polarity-balancing bodywork connects all three main electrical zones during the course of a healing session to ensure the complete flow of energy throughout the entire body. When the body's energy flows freely, the person will be symptom and pain free.

The hands also have specific electrical charges. The right hand has a positive electrical charge, and the left hand has a negative electrical charge. By placing a specific hand on a specific body part—the right hand over a negative-charged body part, or the left hand over a positive-charged body part—the practitioner creates a specific electrical response to clear an energy block.

There are three basic ways to touch the human body, and each one brings about a specific result. The *gentle touch* brings about a sense of well being, balances the nervous system, releases stress, and connects the individual to his spiritual being. An *active touch*, like rocking, stirs the energy. This releases old, stuck energy patterns that have been held in the body so they can change into a new vibrational pattern. The *deep touch* is intense, sometimes painful, and is used to move old, chronic energy patterns that have been held in the body for a very long time.

By understanding the signs of the Zodiac, and the different body parts they correlate to, the practitioner develops a map of the human body. (See Chapter One for the overviews of the chakras and the astrological associations of the first four chakras.) With a completed body-map, the bodyworker knows where to make energy connections to bring about fast and effective results.

. . .

The first chakra is associated with the Earth signs of Taurus, located at the throat; Virgo, located at the bowels; and Capricorn, located at the knees. By connecting these three body parts, neck, bowels, and knees, with the gentle hands-on technique, the earth element and first chakra come into balance.

83

Chapter
Four:
Self
Help
for the
Chakras

To balance the first chakra:

1. Have your client lie on his back on a massage table or futon on the floor. Stand at his right side and place your right hand on your client's right knee, and your left hand on the right side of his navel center. Hold for one minute.

2. Move your left hand to the right side of your client's neck, and your right hand to the right side of his navel center. Hold for one minute.

3. Remain standing at the client's right side, and reverse Steps 1 and 2 on his left side.

• • •

The second chakra is associated with the water signs of Cancer, located in the chest; Scorpio, located at the reproductive system; and Pisces, located at the feet. Connecting these three body parts brings the water element and second chakra into balance.

To balance the second chakra:

1. Have your client lie on his back and stand on the right side. Place your right hand on his right ankle, and your left index finger about two inches above the center of his pubic bone. Massage around the right anklebone for about one minute, while your left finger touches gently. Then hold both contacts gently for another minute.

2. Place your left index finger, about two inches below the mid-collar bone on your client's right side, and your right hand middle finger about two inches above the center of his pubic bone. Hold both contacts for one minute.

2a. Move your left index finger to the center of the chin while keeping your right hand at the center of the pubic bone, and hold for one minute.

2b. Move your left index finger to the center of the forehead (keep your right hand middle finger at the center of the pubic bone), and hold for one minute.

3. Reverse steps 1, 2, 2a, and 2b down the left side of your client's body.

• • •

The third chakra is associated with the fire signs of Aries, located at the head; Leo, located at the solar plexus; and Sagittarius, located at the thighs. Connecting these body parts brings the fire element and third chakra into balance.

To balance the third chakra:
1. Have your client lie on his back and stand at his right side. Place your right hand over his right thigh, and your left hand over his navel center. With your right hand, gently rock up and down the thigh, while your left hand gently rocks the navel center. Do not rock intensely, be gentle and easy. After about thirty seconds of rocking, pause for fifteen seconds, then repeat the rocking once again.

2. Now, place your right hand at your client's navel center, and your left index finger at the inside orbital ridges, where the eyebrows meet above the nose. Hold for about one minute.

3. Reverse steps 1 and 2 on the left side of your client's body.

• • •

The fourth chakra is associated with the air signs of Gemini, located at the chest, shoulders, and arms; Libra, located at the kidneys; and Aquarius, located at the calves and ankles. Connecting these body parts brings the air element and fourth chakra into balance.

To balance the fourth chakra:
1. Have your client lie on his belly and stand on the right. Place your right hand on your client's left calf, and your left hand on his left kidney, located at the bottom of the left rib cage, next to the spine. Massage the left calf down to the left ankle and back to the calf, while the left hand holds at the left kidney. After one minute, hold both contacts without movement.

85

Chapter
Four:
Self
Help
for the
Chakras

2. Place your left hand at your client's left shoulder, and your right hand at your client's left kidney. Hold both contacts for about one minute.

3. Reverse steps 1 and 2 down the right side of your client's body.

4. Stand at your client's head, and place both your hands over the scapulas of the upper back. Hold for about one minute.

• • •

The fifth chakra is associated with the ether element, and is the bridge between the lower physical chakras, and the upper spiritual chakras. The energy of the upper chakras is so subtle, it is beyond the manifestation of the zodiacal signs. The fifth chakra energy correlates to the space of the body and the skeletal system. By balancing the skeletal system, the space of the body is kept clear of energy blocks and the body's structure function flows freely. The three triangular shaped bones that balance the skeletal system are the occiput, sacrum, and heels.

To balance the fifth chakra:
1. Have your client lie on his belly and stand at his right. Place your right hand over your client's sacrum, located where the spine meets the center of the hip, and your left index finger and thumb, on either side of the occiput bone, located where the spine enters the skull. Hold for one minute.

2. Place your left hand over your client's sacrum, and cup your right hand over your client's entire left heel. Hold for thirty seconds, then move your right hand over to your client's right heel. Hold for thirty seconds.

• • •

The sixth chakra's energy correlates to the individual's intuition, psychic awareness, and clairvoyance. This is very spiritual energy accessible only through meditation. The subtle sixth chakra energy appears in the form of visions, pictures, awareness, and knowing.

Balancing the central core, pubic bone, and third eye brings the sixth chakra into balance.

To balance the sixth chakra:

1. Have your client lie on his back and stand on his right. Place the middle finger of your right hand about three inches above the center of your client's pubic bone. Place the index finger of your left hand at the center of the sternum or breastbone. Hold for one minute.

2. Move your left index finger to the center of the chin, and keep the middle finger of your right hand at the center of the pubic bone. Hold for one minute.

3. Move the index finger of your left hand to the center of the forehead (third eye), and keep the middle finger of your right hand at the center of the pubic bone. Hold for one minute.

• • •

The seventh, or crown, chakra energy correlates to the merging of the individual's energy with the universal consciousness. It represents self-realization, and God-realization. By balancing the top of the head, tip of the thumb, and tip of the big toe, the seventh chakra comes into balance.

To balance the seventh chakra:

1. Have your client lie on his back and stand at his right side. Place your left index finger at the top center of the crown. Place the middle finger of your right hand at the center of your client's chin. Hold for one minute.

2. Place the middle finger of your right hand at the tip of your client's right thumb. Keep the index finger of your left hand at the center of the top of your client's head. Hold for one minute.

3. Place the middle finger of your right hand at the tip of your client's right big toe. Place your left index finger at the tip of your client's right thumb. Hold for one minute.

87

Chapter
Four:
Self
Help
for the
Chakras

4. Reverse steps 1, 2, and 3 on the other side of your client's body.

• • •

The polarity balancing healing system is a wonderful way to help people, help themselves. It is gentle, loving, respectful, and kind.

Understanding Karma with Astrology

The physical body is comprised of divine energy, classified into the cosmic five-element theory. Each element correlates to a different body energy system: ether, associated with the nervous system; air, associated with the respiratory and circulatory systems; fire, associated with the digestive system; water, associated with the reproductive system; and earth, associated with the excretory system. The only difference between the cosmic five elements is the different rates of speed at which they vibrate. One element is not better than another element. Each element manifests divine energy in a different way, thus creating the different energy systems of the body.

Besides correlating to the physical body, the cosmic five elements also correlate to the individual's personality, tendencies, attributes, likes, dislikes, etc. The cosmic five elements manifest differently in each individual according to the karmic lessons she must learn from previous lifetimes, and from the choices she makes in this lifetime. The theory of karma states that the desired result for all human beings is to clear all negative action and become one with God consciousness. Karma is action in life. Every individual action, whether positive or negative, creates karma. Negative karma keeps the individual attached to her body. Positive karma sets her soul free of the cycle of birth and death, and she does not have to reincarnate back into a physical body. In order to accomplish the goal of clearing negative karma, the individual must purify his spiritual, mental, emotional, and physical beings by learning lessons in life. Each lesson offers an opportunity for growth, and it is up to the individual to recognize the opportunity, learn her lesson, and clear her karma.

Clearing karma is a transformational process that can take many years of searching and personal growth. Often, clearing negative karma is not accomplished in one lifetime. The individual must then reincarnate to continue the healing process. The unresolved lessons from past lives come along into the new lifetime so the individual can complete his journey. Sometimes the healing process can take many, many lifetimes.

Each time the individual is born into a body, the law of karma is in effect. The law of karma determines how the planets are aligned during the exact moment of the individual's birth. Karma also determines the individual's sex, place of birth, who the individual's parents and other family members are, the individual's zodiacal sign, etc. By understanding the zodiac, and what kinds of behavioral tendencies may occur with each sign, people can gain a better understanding of who they are. This will assist in clearing karmic lessons.

The Twelve Signs of the Zodiac

There are twelve zodiacal signs in astrology, three for each of the four cardinal elements.

The three Earth signs are Taurus, Virgo, and Capricorn.

A Taurus person, born from April 20th to May 20th, moves slowly, needs time to adjust to new ideas, and is stubborn. She has a strong desire for job security, and to maintain a secure home. She loves to acquire material things, and enjoys the comfort of plush surroundings. She is deeply driven to obtain a rich life style, and is not afraid to go after what she wants no matter the cost.

A Virgo, born from August 22nd to September 22nd, has a strong desire to be perfect. He loves to organize, and is concerned about the details of his job, home, and creative projects. He enjoys being home, and has a down to earth, practical approach to life. The Virgo person loves to analyze everything, with a tendency to become overly critical. He is generally quiet, and makes friends easily. He is also very healthy, and will go to great lengths to maintain good health.

89

Chapter
Four:
Self
Help
for the
Chakras

A Capricorn, born from December 20th to January 21st, has a strong sense of purpose and is determined to accomplish her goals. She is ambitious and willing to put forth her best effort to succeed. The Capricorn person is a leader, dependable in her work habits, with the energy and willingness to help others. Money, power, and success are extremely important to Capricorns, who love the challenge of overcoming adversity to accomplish a goal.

The three water signs are Cancer, Scorpio, and Pisces.

The Cancer person, born from June 21st to July 21st, responds to life through his emotions. He has strong feelings about everything. Sometimes he absorbs the feelings of others, and vacillates up and down with intense mood swings. It is difficult for him to be direct, and he may sidestep issues. The Cancer person is very intuitive and can easily respond to the psychic energy of others. He becomes very attached to people, places, and things and when he gives his heart in love, it is forever. The Cancer individual loves his home and taking care of it. At the first sign of trouble, he wants to return to the safety of his home. He also enjoys nurturing others and providing a safe, emotional space to process feelings.

The Scorpio individual, born from October 21st to November 22nd, is mysterious in nature and likes to be alone. She is quiet and introspective. Making friends is a process because of the Scorpio intensity. The person can easily scare people away because of an abundance of creative energy. If someone falls out of favor with a Scorpio, there will probably be a confrontation. A Scorpio has a razor sharp tongue, and can be rude, sarcastic, and mean-spirited when feeling threatened. A Scorpio individual has strong passions and loves sex. She is at her best when serving others.

The Pisces person, born from February 21st to March 21st, is the most sensitive among the signs. A Pisces is moody, inward, and difficult to understand. He needs alone time to reconnect with his inner being. Once he finds balance with his inner being, he only wants to serve humankind. He has great compassion for all people of the world. A Piscean has a tremendous amount of creativity that needs to be channeled through the arts.

The three fire signs are Aries, Leo, and Sagittarius.

The Aries person, born from March 21st to April 21st, is wonderful at getting projects started. She is always willing to create new ways to break through any obstruction that might be in the way of her accomplishing a goal. The Aries individual has a lot of energy and is confident in whatever she does. She likes to be busy all the time, and to have things done her way. She does not like her life to be complicated with unnecessary details, and gets bored easily. Relaxation is important in teaching the individual how to conserve energy.

The Leo individual, born from July 21st to August 22nd, has dignity, self-respect, courage, and integrity. The Leo person is honest and direct and brings joy to others through altruistic endeavors. A Leo person likes to be in charge of people, places, and things. Sometimes he has difficulty in giving up power and attempts to do everything by himself. This behavior is draining and could lead to health problems. A Leo person always wants to do the right thing. Once he falls in love, he will love forever.

The Sagittarius individual, born from November 21st to December 21st, is friendly, outgoing, optimistic, and independent. She needs room and does not like to be fenced in. The Sagittarian values freedom and loves to travel. She is straightforward and does not procrastinate. She sets goals and does whatever she needs to do to accomplish them. A Sagittarian has lots of energy for all the things she likes to do, and moves from one project to another easily.

The three air signs are Gemini, Libra, and Aquarius.

The Gemini person, individual, born from May 21st to June 21st, may be a good teacher, writer, thinker, and communicator. He makes friends easily and enjoys all kinds of relationships. A Gemini moves easily from one group of people to another. He enjoys many different types of stimuli, keeping his mind busy. The Gemini individual has a tendency to focus too much on mental activities and could

91

Chapter
Four:
Self
Help
for the
Chakras

exhaust himself from doing too much. His nervous system can stress easily, so he has to rest and be still for periods of time. Geminis have many different types of personalities, which make them interesting people to interact with.

The Libra person, born from September 21st to October 21st, is friendly, outgoing, and desires to live life to the fullest. She sees herself as an ambassador of good will, and has a strong desire to be liked by everyone. A Libra is the peacemaker of the zodiac, and she seeks balance in all relationships and things. She may be a great negotiator and caregiver. A Libra likes to travel and see the world. She does not like to be inside a house for too long and will have a difficult time if she is confined to one area.

The Aquarius person, born from January 21st to February 22nd, is outgoing, friendly, and has a tremendous amount of confidence. He is a thinker and loves to spend time in the future, not dwelling on the past. He is an intellectual, who thrives in the sciences and arts, and loves to write. He enjoys serving others, and he receives tremendous satisfaction when involved with humanitarian deeds. An Aquarian is extremely strong-willed, and can be difficult to get along with. Aquarians are born leaders and are not afraid to break ground with new ideas and concepts.

The Ten Heavenly Bodies

Another major influence upon the individual's karma is how the energies of the planets line up in his astrological chart. The different energies of the planets correspond to different energies available to the individual, affecting the choices one makes. By understanding these different energies the individual can be influenced to use the right course of action to achieve his goals.

The Sun's energy integrates all of life's lessons, and helps the individual achieve his goals. Sun energy gives one the power to do, the power to be, and correlates to the life force energy or *prana*. The life force energy rules all beings: spiritual, mental, emotional, and physical. The Sun's placement in the individual's birth chart indicates where that person will be able to excel in life. The Sun rules Leo and the third chakra.

The Moon's energy helps one to love all people and to receive love from others. Moon energy keeps the individual in touch with his feelings. Emotional ups and downs are ruled by Moon energy. The ability to nurture others and understand the feelings of others is also ruled by Moon energy. Moon energy helps the individual feel the subtle energy of the Earth, especially when the Earth experiences energetic changes. Moon energy manifestation in the birth chart indicates the individual's emotional being. The Moon rules Cancer and the second chakra.

Mercury energy rules the intellect. It is the link between the physical and spiritual beings. All communication, internally or externally, is governed by Mercury. Mercury energy assists with the understanding of complex ideas and universal concepts, expanding universal consciousness and the ability to help humankind. Mercury energy's manifestation in the birth chart indicates what new techniques and skills are needed to continue the learning process. Mercury rules Gemini and the fourth chakra; and Virgo and the first chakra. Because it is the bridge between the physical and mental beings, it also rules the fifth chakra.

Venus energy helps the individual open to universal love energy. When the individual truly believes in universal love and lives his life loving others regardless of what others do or say, he has immersed himself in Venus energy. When the individual lives through his spiritual convictions, and loves all people, places and things, he has discovered the essence of Venus energy. Venus's manifestation in the birth chart indicates where universal love energy needs to be integrated into the person's life. Venus rules Taurus and the first chakra; and Libra, and the fourth chakra.

Mars energy bursts forth with enthusiasm, and gives the energy to do things and accomplish goals in life. Mars energy is the spark of life, and gives one the perseverance to complete projects. Mars energy can be overpowering, and it might appear that the individual is attempting to control others. Sometimes, people have a difficult time being around an upbeat Mars person. Mars energy is masculine and outgoing. Mars energy manifestation in the birth chart indicates where there is a store-

93

Chapter
Four:
Self
Help
for the
Chakras

house of energy available that the individual must pay attention to. If this energy is not channeled properly, it could bring chaos. Mars rules Aries and the third chakra; and Scorpio and the second chakra.

Saturn energy is very focused and concentrated. It indicates where an individual needs to make changes in his life so he can progress and clear his negative energy. Saturn energy allows the individual to bring new concepts and new awareness to current attitudes that need changing. Saturn energy gives the individual the ability to move forward in life, transforming stuck negative energy into new-found courage, strength, and determination. Saturn energy manifestation in the birth chart indicates where the individual must begin the journey to create new structures in life. Saturn rules Capricorn and the first chakra; and Aquarius and the fourth chakra.

Jupiter energy represents the individual's connection to the universal love energy. It rules the individual's super consciousness, giving the energy to open up to the higher principles and ideals of life. When the universal principles of love are grasped, one can make new choices to better oneself and humankind. In the spiritual aspects of life Jupiter energy is very expansive, giving the individual a strong sense of faith to carry through any difficult situation. Jupiter manifestation in the birth chart is where the individual will receive fulfillment. Jupiter rules Sagittarius and the third chakra; and because it correlates to spiritual awareness, Jupiter rules the sixth and seventh chakras as well.

Uranus energy is the individual's link to cosmic consciousness. Uranus energy opens the individual's mind to universal knowledge, and his heart to universal love. When the individual gains insight to universal truth, he can use his relationship with the truth to assist humankind. Uranus energy allows the individual to connect with the universal truth, and trust intuition, so he can relax, wait, and respond to the subtle energy changes of the Earth in a centered way, and adjust to whatever energy changes the universe provides. Wherever Uranus manifests in the birth chart is where the individual must surrender to his higher power and let the cosmic forces rule. Uranus rules Aquarius and the fourth chakra; and because of its direct link to cosmic consciousness, it rules the seventh chakra.

Neptune energy allows the individual to wander into the psychic realms and enter into other energetic dimensions. The individual dreams through Neptune: dreams of other worlds, dreams of the other lifetimes, dreams of the unknown. Neptune allows the individual to see what others cannot see, to visualize what others cannot envision, and to know what others cannot know. With Neptune energy the individual's feelings are enhanced, and her imagination soars. Sometimes Neptune energy is so airy it can be difficult for the individual to be present in the physical world. Wherever Neptune energy manifests in the birth chart indicates where the individual must serve. When the individual serves humankind, many benefit. Neptune rules Pisces and the second chakra; and since our psychic abilities are enhanced, Neptune rules the sixth chakra.

Pluto energy assists the individual in transforming his dense, heavy, old negative patterns, into new patterns that support his connection to spirit. By using Pluto energy, the individual can easily let go of the past and become one with the cosmic consciousness. Pluto energy helps the individual to change, rediscover feelings, and bring forth new ideas. It brings hope to the individual and renews his sense of who he really is. Wherever Pluto energy manifests in the birth chart indicates that part of the individual that must be reborn. Pluto rules Aries and the third chakra; Scorpio, the second chakra; and the sixth and seventh chakras.

The Twelve Houses

In astrology, each house represents a certain type of energy. When the birth chart is read, an individual can observe what planets reside in what house. Since the planets also correspond to certain energy qualities, observing what planet is in what house will indicate many of the tendencies or lessons that the individual will be faced with during his lifetime. This information can assist a person in making choices to best achieve his goals.

First house energy reflects one's outlook on life. What are her likes or dislikes? How will these affect her course of action? What is necessary for her to be happy? How is she going to lead her life? Does

95

Chapter
Four:
Self
Help
for the
Chakras

she like the way she looks and acts? The first house correlates to the first chakra.

Second house energy reflects the individual's attitudes about material possessions and money. How much money does he need to have before he feels secure? Does he measure success through business and financial gain? Does he need to own a big house before he feels happy? Does he think that happiness occurs through the material world? If he identifies his existence through the physical world of money and possessions, it will lead to unhappiness. The second house correlates to the second chakra.

Third house energy reflects the individual's attitudes toward the environment, other family members, neighbors, and people in general. Is she happy with her circle of friends? Do they support her emotionally and mentally? Does she see herself as part of her local community? Is his local community part of the world community? How do world events affect him? The third house correlates to the third chakra.

Fourth house energy reflects the relationship the individual has between the physical world and his inner world. Can the individual move between both worlds with harmony and ease? Would it be in the best interest of the individual to branch out into the physical world or stay home? Can he make the transition? What will happen to him if he chooses to be inward or outward? Can he live in both worlds? How does he define his environment? The fourth house correlates to the first chakra.

Fifth house energy reflects the uniqueness of the individual. How is the individual different from others? What type of work does she like to do? What are her special interests? How does she feel about family, children, and relationships? How does the individual express herself, especially when it comes to matters of the heart? How is love and romance manifesting in her life? The fifth house correlates to the second and fourth chakras.

Sixth house energy reflects the individual's ability to serve humankind without any regard for reward, or karma yoga. There is no attachment to the finished product and all action is undertaken while thinking of spirit. Sixth house energy also correlates with the ability of the individual to take care of himself. Can he work hard without overextending himself? Can he pace himself so he won't get run down? Sixth house energy allows the person to spread joy throughout the community. The sixth house correlates to the fifth chakra.

Seventh house energy reflects the individual's ability to have successful relationships in business and family. Is the individual determined enough to overcome any obstacles that might interfere with maintaining harmony in these relationships? Can she cooperate with others? Does she have the ability to move forward in a mature way? Can she overcome the challenges of having a big ego? Does she see the whole picture when it comes to the needs and wants of others? The seventh house correlates to the second chakra.

Eighth house energy reflects the individual's ability to help humankind by taking a stance against injustices brought about by greed and avarice. The individual knows that if the general population does not change its attitudes toward material gain and profit seeking, the world will suffer greater consequences in the future. It is important for her to hold true to her convictions and help humankind shift its consciousness toward loving one another. The eighth house correlates to the sixth chakra.

Ninth house energy reflects the individual's ability to use his spiritual energy to understand who he really is. When he relies on his intuition, his choices in life come from his soul. By living from his soul he is always in harmony with spirit. By being in harmony with spirit, he truly understands his mental, emotional, and physical beings. His horizons are expanded to new levels of awareness and he can experience oneness with all things. The ninth house correlates to the sixth and seventh chakras.

Tenth house energy reflects the choices the individual makes with regard to career opportunities, and how society views her type of work. Is she acting with integrity in her work? Does her work have a positive impact on society? Is she just working to earn money? Does she want to work in a field that serves humankind? Does she feel

97

Chapter
Four:
Self
Help
for the
Chakras

worthy of working a job that assists others? Does she have the energy to help others? Is she concerned about payment for her work? The tenth house correlates to the second and fifth chakras.

Eleventh house energy reflects the hopes, dreams, and desires that the individual has about life. How are his relationships and friendships manifesting? Is he finding happiness with others easily, or does it take a lot of effort? Do other people care about him and do they want to be associated with him? What are his long-term goals in business and relationships? How does he see himself in relationship to the rest of the world? Where does he fit into society? The individual's consciousness is heightened in this house, enabling him to better express his intellect and emotions. The eleventh house correlates to the second and fourth chakras.

Twelfth house energy reflects the ability of the individual to sacrifice her wants and desires for the benefit of others. She knows that spirit will take care of her, so she does not need to put herself first. It is her conscious choice to serve others and by doing so, she surrenders completely to spirit, and she can clear her past negative karma. Before she can unite with spirit, she must let go of all the hidden wants and desires of the mind. As she surrenders, she becomes clear. The twelfth house correlates to the sixth and seventh chakras.

• • •

A person's astrological sign and horoscope are the blueprint of his life. It describes how the universal energy will effect him, why he was born, and the lessons he has to learn to free himself of his negative karma. The planets indicate what his wants and desires are, and describe the energies available to him to accomplish his goals. The houses show him where to go to find out what his lessons are; they are the situations that develop that give opportunities for growth.

Mantras

Mantras are ancient Sanskrit phrases that carry the cosmic universal love energy. The repetition of the mantra creates a positive energy field. Each mantra has a specific vibrational code attached to it. There are mantras to help humankind come into balance with all aspects of life, for protection, for healing, to improve digestion, to improve vision, to achieve peace, to achieve happiness, to heal from snake bites, to change the weather, to achieve mental clarity, and many other purposes.

The ancient yogis and *rishis* (seers) of India realized how to access the human energy fields through the use of sound. It was this understanding that helped develop the ancient language of Sanskrit, a most unusual language designed to carry the vibrational essence of the cosmic universal love energy. It was not developed for commerce, trade, or to express the everyday things in life. Instead, its major focus is to convey the spiritual essence of the cosmic universal love energy in all of its expressions.

As mantras are chanted, a positive energy is created. The more often the individual repeats a mantra, the easier it is to change negative energy into positive energy. Once the subtle energy fields are cleared of all negativity, it is easier for the individual to manifest the cosmic universal love energy into his everyday life.

When Mahatma Gandhi's son was stricken with typhoid fever, Gandhi refused all medicines and simply chanted the mantra, *"Shri Rama Jai Rama Jay Jay Ram."* Gandhi's devotion to the power of mantras was strong, and shortly after he began chanting the mantra, his son was completely healed of the disease. There are literally thousands of true stories like Gandhi's that document the healing power of mantras.

It is recommended that an individual develop a relationship with the mantras he intends to use. In this way, the mantras will become part of his life, and when it is necessary for him to use them, he will be familiar with them. Just understanding how to say the mantras is not good enough. It is recommended that the individual sit in meditation and practice the recitation of the mantras daily for at least one month, before using them. The minimum number of repetitions of the mantra during meditation is one hundred and eight. Chanting with *mala* beads can be used to keep track of how many times the mantra has been said during meditation. The mala has one

99

Chapter
Four:
Self
Help
for the
Chakras

hundred and eight beads on a string. One time around the mala beads will complete the cycle for the day. If there is more time available, continue chanting the mantras for the remainder of time allowed for that day. The more the individual chants the mantras, the deeper her relationship will be with them. By developing a deep relationship with the mantras, when the time comes to use the mantras for balancing or healing, they will work.

Another benefit received from chanting the mantras is that the individual will have the opportunity to heal herself of any imbalances that she has created within her body, mind, and spirit. She will feel peaceful, content, lighter, softer, and in harmony with all beings. Her agitated mind will become quiet; her emotions will become balanced, and she will feel more connected to spirit. Once the individual begins to chant mantras, it could become part of her daily life.

Mantras to Balance the Seven Chakras

The first chakra

Om Shri Ganeshaya Namaha.
Salutations to Lord Ganesha, the remover of all obstacles.

The second chakra

Shri Rama Jaya Rama Jaya Jaya Rama.
Salutations to Lord Ram, conqueror of lust and greed.

The third chakra

Om Eim Saraswati Namaha.
Saraswati, bless me with clear mental intentions.

The fourth chakra

Om Vamanaya Namaha.
Salutations to Vamana, bless me with humility and virtues.

The fifth chakra

Om Shri Hanumate Namaha.
Blessings to Hanuman, who blesses us with victory over all things.

The sixth chakra
Om Eim Hreem Kleem Chamundayai Viche Namaha.
Blessings to Shakti, who gives us wisdom and power.

The seventh chakra
So Ham Hansaha Swaha.
I am He, He is me, we are one together.
Om Shanti, Shanti, Shanti.
Om peace, peace, peace.

• • •

The following are mantras to cultivate strength and overcome negative tendencies:

To cultivate courage and strength chant the mantra:
Sita, Rama, Sita, Rama, Gurudeva Hare, Hare.
I surrender to Sita and Rama.

To celebrate life and rejoice, chant the mantra:
Sarvah Sarvatra Nandatu.
Let everyone everywhere rejoice.

For health and happiness, chant the mantra:
Sarve Bhavantu Sukhinah, Sarve Santu Niramayaha.
In everything let them be happy, let them be healthy.

To cultivate oneness with God, chant the mantra:
Om Nama Shivaya. Lord Shiva.
I surrender to you.

To cultivate prosperity in your life, chant the mantra,
Om Lakshmi Namaha.
I honor you Lakshmi, Goddess of prosperity.

To bring happiness to all peoples chant:
Lokaha Samastaha Sukeenu Bavantu.

101

Chapter
Four:
Self
Help
for the
Chakras

· · ·

There are hundreds of mantras designed to assist the healing the individual in healing his body, mind, and spirit; I have mentioned just a few. Be devoted in your practice of the mantras, and they will assist you in becoming one with everything.

Homeopathy

Homeopathy was discovered by Dr. Samuel Hahnemann in the early 1800s. Homeopathy is based on the law of similars. The law of similars states that a natural remedy can cure any disease if the remedy brings about symptoms of the disease in a healthy person. Simply stated, like cures like.

In practice, the law of homeopathy works this way. When an individual becomes sick, she might develop symptoms such as a runny nose, cough with a rattle, and a slight headache. The homeopathic practitioner studies all of the symptoms, then looks for a homeopathic remedy that will bring about the same symptoms in a healthy person. Hopefully, after the sick person takes the remedy, her symptoms will disappear and she will recover.

Homeopathic remedies are prepared from plants, minerals, flowers, roots, animals, insects, and reptiles. The item that is going to be used to make a remedy is soaked in alcohol for two weeks beginning on the new moon. Two weeks later, on the full moon, the alcohol is strained off and becomes the mother tincture. To make a 1C potency remedy, place one drop of the mother tincture and ninety-nine drops of purified water or alcohol in a bottle. Shake the bottle vigorously thirty times. To continue making higher dosage C potencies, take one drop of the 1C potency remedy and add ninety-nine drops of purified water or alcohol in a bottle. Shake vigorously thirty times. This will give you a 2C potency remedy. Continue this process for all higher dosage C remedies. Once you reach 12C potency, all the physical properties of the remedy are removed and what remains is the vibrational essence of the remedy. The higher the dosage, the stronger the remedy. Health food stores sell remedies up to 30C potency.

To make a 1X potency remedy, take one drop of the mother tincture and add to it nine drops of purified water or alcohol in a bottle. Shake vigorously thirty times. To continue making higher dosage X remedies, take one drop of the 1X remedy, add nine drops of purified water or alcohol in a bottle. Shake the bottle vigorously thirty times. This will give you a 2X remedy. Continue this process for all higher dosage X remedies. Once you reach 24X potency, all the physical properties of the remedy are removed and what remains is the vibrational essence of the remedy. The higher the dosage, the stronger the remedy. Health food stores sell remedies up to 30X potency. When all of the physical properties are diluted out of the original remedy, it is considered a high potency remedy. When some of the physical properties remain in the original remedy, it is a low potency remedy. The higher the dilution of the remedy, the greater the healing effect upon the body. Sometimes it is recommended that the healing be slow and easy with the client, so a lower dosage remedy will serve the client better than a more powerful one. So it is up to the homeopathic practitioner to determine the correct dosage and remedy for the client

Since homeopathic remedies are so subtle and work with the individual's vibrational essence, there are certain rules that are recommended to ensure that the remedies will work once taken internally.

Do not place the pills in your hand. Homeopathic remedies come in the form of tiny sugar pills. The sugar pills have been coated with the liquid form of the remedy. By placing the pills in your hand, the oils, salts, and sweat of your hand can negate the effectiveness of the remedy. Shake the pills into the lid of the container that they are packaged in, and put them under your tongue. Do not chew the pills, let them dissolve. You can also dissolve the pills in a glass of water, and sip the water slowly.

Do not drink any liquid for fifteen minutes before or after you take any remedy.

Only take one remedy at a time, to ensure you know which remedy is working for what symptom.

Chapter
Four:
Self
Help
for the
Chakras

Do not drink coffee or any caffeinated drink during the day you take any remedy. This could negate the effect of the remedy.

Stay away from strong smelling substances like peppermint, camphor, basil, or spices when you are planning to take any remedy. These could negate the effectiveness of the remedy.

Homeopathic medicine really works. It is a wonderful way to help people help themselves. The remedies work on an inner core, and assist the body's immune system to function at optimum capacity. There are no side effects from any of the remedies, and the remedies can assist both acute and chronic ailments and symptoms.

Homeopathic Remedies to Balance the seven chakras

The first chakra: Aconitum Napellus, Alumina (also used for Alzheimer's disease).

The second chakra: Hepar Sulphur, Calcareum.

The third chakra: Nux Vomica, Ipecacuanha, Carbo Vegetabilis.

The fourth chakra: Phosophorus, Spongia Tosta, Histaminum.

The fifth chakra: Mercurius Solubilius, Pulsatilla.

The sixth chakra: Ignatia Amara, Coffea, Aurum Metticulum.

The seventh chakra: Chamomilla, Hyoscyamus, Sulphur.

Homeopathic Remedies for Common Ailments and Complaints

Bee stings or bug bites: Apis Mellifica.

Physical trauma, sprains, bruises, muscular aches: Arnica Montana.

Rapid development of symptoms, flushed face: Belladona.

Minor burns, blistering, itching: Cantharis.

Headache: Ignatia Amara.

Puncture wound: Ledum Palustre.

Allergies: Histaminum.

Bleeding: Cinchona Officinalis.

Anxiety: Aconitum Napellus.

Diarrhea: Ipecacuanha, Colocynthis.

Eye strain: Ruta Graveolens.
Indigestion: Carbo Vegetabilis.
Menstrual cramps: Magnesia Phosphoricum.
Nausea: Ipecacuanha.
Sunburn: Canatharis.
Joint pain: Byronia.
Constipation: Alumina.

There are thousands of homeopathic remedies available. Consult with your local homeopathic physician or practitioner for best results. I recommend the book, Homeopathic Vibrations, by David Dancu. This is a wonderful book that will assist you in understanding how homeopathy works.

Diet

Diet plays an extremely important role in health and longevity. What to eat, when to eat it, where to eat, whom to eat with, what foods to combine are valid questions about diet that need to be answered. When an individual takes responsibility for his own healing, he begins to listen to his inner intuitive voice that is always giving him information about himself. By listening, he can respond with his truth in all situations, and his intuition will give him the information he needs to know about his diet. When the individual consumes food due to mental, emotional, or spiritual stress, the physical body will have difficulty digesting it. This can lead to physical imbalances or blocks in the person's energy fields.

All foods consumed are classified within the first, second, third, and fourth chakras. The fifth, sixth, and seventh chakras are vibrating at such a high rate of speed, foods are not classified to them. Foods correlate to the chakras according to how and where they grow.

Foods that grow underground like beets, carrots, turnips, parsnips, and potatoes, are classified with the first chakra. Please note: Foods like ginger, garlic, and onions, are the exception because although they grow underground, their heating properties are so great that they are classified under the third chakra.

105

Chapter
Four:
Self
Help
for the
Chakras

Foods that grow on the surface of the ground like leafy green vegetables (lettuce, spinach), beans, mushrooms, radishes, parsley, cucumbers, squash, celery, peppers, eggplants, melons, cabbage, and cauliflower are classified with the second chakra.

Foods that grow from two to eight feet above the ground like barley, wheat, corn, oats, rye, rice, millet, quinoa, and aramath are classified under the third chakra.

Foods that grow high in trees like, lemons, limes, grapefruits, pears, apples, peaches, nectarines, plums, cherries, coconuts, apricots, and figs are classified with the fourth chakra.

Eating foods from each chakra classification, will balance the person's energy. Forming proper eating habits will result in optimum digestion.

Common Sense about Eating

Only eat when you are sitting down. Walking down the street while eating food, will make the food indigestible.

Avoid eating quickly. If you don't have enough time to complete your meal, don't eat. Wait until you have more time so you won't be interrupted.

Avoid distractions while you eat. Making phone calls or watching television while you are eating will result in poor digestion.

Avoid eating when you are angry. Food can't be digested while you are emotionally upset.

Stop eating before you feel full. Don't continue eating because the food tastes good. This will lead to overeating and poor digestion.

Eat food when you are hungry and drink liquids when you are thirsty. If you eat when you are thirsty, and drink when you are hungry, your entire digestive system will be out of balance resulting in gas, poor digestion, and constipation.

Bless your food before you eat it. Blessing the food changes its vibrational essence and makes the food easier to digest. This is especially true in restaurants because you do not know the state of mind of all the people preparing and handling the food. Blessing the food removes any negativity and improves digestion.

Proper food selection is learned through trial and error. The thing to remember is that the right food for one individual isn't always right for someone else. There are no set rules. The individual's age, constitution, temperament, and capabilities for digesting and assimilating food are all factors in determining what foods are best suited for him. Acknowledge these factors to establish a balanced diet. It is up to the individual to take the time to figure out what the best choices are.

About Meals

Simple meals are most easily digested. Eating a wide variety of foods at one sitting confuses the enzyme-producing organs, which then produce the wrong kinds or amounts of digestive juices.

Digestion begins in the mouth. All solid food should be well-chewed and mixed with saliva. Most people don't chew their food enough, resulting in slowed digestion and assimilation.

Eat meals slowly. When a person eats too fast, there is no consciousness about the food or the amount being consumed. This leads to overeating.

Food Combinations

Understanding what happens to food as it is being digested will help an individual make a conscious choice of what foods to eat. The following food combinations should be avoided because they slow down the digestive process:

Starches and Proteins. When starch foods like potatoes, wheat, rice, corn, oats, are combined with proteins like meats or beans, digestion is slowed. Both types of food require different types of enzymes for proper digestion. Starches are digested by the alkaline enzymes found in the mouth and small intestine. Proteins are digested by the acid enzymes found in the stomach. The acid enzymes of the stomach destroy the alkaline enzymes from the mouth, so the starches that began digestion in the mouth are greatly slowed when they enter the stomach. This causes indigestion and gas. When whole foods containing both starches and proteins are consumed by themselves, the stomach does not produce its acid-forming enzymes to digest the protein until the starches have been completely digested by the alkaline enzymes of the mouth.

107

Chapter
Four:
Self
Help
for the
Chakras

Starches and Acidic Foods. The acid found in citrus fruits like oranges, lemons, limes, and grapefruits destroys the alkaline enzymes needed to properly digest starches. The starches then ferment, causing excess gas, a bloated feeling, and indigestion.

Starches and Sugars. When starches are consumed with sugars, the sugar stops the secretion of the alkaline enzymes needed to digest the starches. This results in fermentation. The constant consumption of cakes, donuts, and pastries will lead to indigestion, increased weight gain, feeling bloated, and poor assimilation.

Proteins and Acidic Foods. When acidic foods like citrus fruits, tomatoes, and vinegar are consumed with proteins, they stop the flow of digestive enzymes in the stomach, and prevent the proteins from being digested.

Proteins. Every protein requires a specific digestive enzyme for proper digestion. If you consume more than one protein at a meal, it becomes difficult for the body to produce all the specific enzymes necessary to digest the different proteins. As a result, digestion is slowed.

Proteins and Fats. When fats like margarine, butter, or cooking oils are consumed with proteins like nuts, meats, or eggs, the fats stop the flow of enzymes that digest the proteins. As a result, digestion is slowed.

Proteins and Sugars. When sugars and proteins are consumed, the sugars slow down the flow of enzymes that digest proteins. Proteins are digested first, with the sugars waiting to be digested afterwards. This results in fermentation and slowed digestion.

The following of food combinations will ensure proper digestion and assimilation.

- Vegetables and proteins combine well together.
- Vegetables and starches combine well together.
- Sweet fruits like bananas and dates are best eaten alone.
- Fruits that contain a high level of acid like citrus or tomatoes are best eaten alone.
- Combining partially acidic fruits like apricots, berries, plums, and peaches with sweet fruits is all right.
- Any type of melon is best consumed by itself.

• • •

Food selection and food combining is an individual choice. If you suffer from any digestive difficulty, closely monitoring food combinations will greatly assist you in fine tuning your eating patterns. This is only a guideline to discovering what to eat to avoid indigestion. It is up to you to think about the types of foods you consume, how you combine them, and to make healthy choices.

Things to Remember while Eating

Food is digested in layers. The first thing eaten will be the first thing digested.

Don't be fooled by processed or chemicalized food. They can trick you into overeating because they are readily prepared and taste so good. These foods are usually eaten quickly, with little regard for caloric intake. As a result, the body receives a surplus of calories without receiving any nutritional value.

Eat organic foods as much as possible. This will cut down on the amount of chemicals and pesticides ingested.

If the food does not taste good, do not eat it. The digestive juices will not flow properly and the food will be poorly digested.

When you see, smell, and taste food, the body begins to secrete digestive enzymes. If the food is disguised with different sauces, preservatives and chemicals, the digestive system doesn't know how to react. This causes poor digestion. When digestive dysfunction is repeated over a long period of time, the body may manifest disease.

Improper eating patterns lead to diseases of the body. Think about what you eat, when you eat it. Eat with love and stop eating before you are full. A balanced diet of 30 percent grains, 20 percent protein, 40 percent fresh fruits and vegetables, 5 percent nuts and seeds, and 5 percent fat enables the individual to maintain a healthy body, and keep his bodily systems working efficiently.

Angelic Affirmations

Angelic affirmations are a wonderful way to clear the mind of any unwanted, negative mental vibrational patterns. These negative men-

109

Chapter
Four:
Self
Help
for the
Chakras

tal patterns create a negative outlook of the world and a negative reality in the day-to-day events of life. Having a negative response to events and experiences becomes a bad habit that can be difficult to change.

The negative mental and emotional reaction to events and situations is a learned behavioral response. The individual learned this type of behavior from his primary care-givers early in life. He didn't just wake up one day and become negative in his outlook of life, it was instilled into his value system. While growing up, if the messages he heard from his primary caregivers were negative, his outlook on life will be negative. There is no getting around this, regardless of how he rationalizes his experience. Sometimes this is difficult to acknowledge because he wants to believe that he was raised by loving parents in a loving household. Often, this is not the case. Changing the mental perspective from a negative outlook to a positive outlook is the first step in healing the old, negative mental patterns.

Angelic affirmations can assist a person in becoming positive in their mental outlook. Angelic affirmations change the negative mental vibrational patterns, into clear, positive mental responses. They are fun, easy to do, and positive results will come quickly.

The easiest way to use the angelic affirmations is to sit quietly in a comfortable position, then determine which chakra is out of balance or needs work. After determining which chakra is to be cleared of negativity, meditate on that chakra with the appropriate angelic affirmation. Repeat the affirmation three times.

Angelic affirmation to balance the first chakra.

Sit in a comfortable position and place your hands in your lap with your palms open. Imagine a beam of golden light dropping like a stone from the base of your spine, deep into the center of the Earth.
Affirmation: I am one with the Earth, where I receive nurturing, courage, and strength.

Angelic affirmation to balance the second chakra.

Sit in a comfortable position and place your hands below your navel center, above the pubic bone. Feel the creative force of the universe flowing through you like a stream flowing down a hillside.

Affirmation: I am one with balance, harmony, and the creative power of God.

Angelic affirmation to balance the third chakra.
Sit in a comfortable position and place your hands on your navel center. Imagine the pure golden light of the Sun, radiating from you.
Affirmation: I am one with the power of God's love, and I radiate this love into my world.

Angelic affirmation to balance the fourth chakra.
Sit in a comfortable position and place your hands on your heart. Breathe in the warmth of the universe.
Affirmation: I am one with radiant health and beauty.

Angelic affirmation to balance the fifth chakra.
Sit in a chair, with palms together, and place your hands to your throat. Feel the vastness of the universe, ever expanding.
Affirmation: I am one with the clear expression of God's truth, wisdom, and compassion.

Angelic affirmation to balance the sixth chakra.
Sit in a comfortable position with palms together, place your hands to your forehead. Feel the white light of the universe coming into your being.
Affirmation: I am one with clarity and wisdom.

Angelic affirmation to balance the seventh chakra.
Sit in a comfortable position and place your palms together in a prayer position above your head. Connect with the universal love energy coming into your entire being through the crown,
Affirmation: I am one with the supreme power, the source of all life.

Angelic affirmations to uplift your spirits and enhance your personal growth:

To cultivate spiritual awareness: Ask to be a receptacle for pure light, then allow the empty chalice within you to drink the sweetness that is God's love.

111

Chapter
Four:
Self
Help
for the
Chakras

To cultivate trust: Trust in the universal flow of good and know there is a perfect outworking in all situations.

To cultivate high self-esteem: Accept that you are a radiant spirit of light who is growing stronger everyday in patterns of wholeness and truth.

To cultivate right action: When you dedicate your life to God, you move into the life stream of pure consciousness where there are no limitations.

To cultivate intuition: Resonate with what is true for you and leave the rest.

To cultivate knowledge: Be aware that the answers to all you are seeking are within you.

To cultivate prosperity: All the money I give is blessed and returned to me multiplied.

To cultivate responsibility: You attract to you only that which is in your consciousness.

To cultivate assistance: Call on us often and picture the wings of angels enfolding you in light.

To cultivate acceptance: All that you have learned and all that has happened to you, brought you to where you are now. Be grateful.

To cultivate love: One way to balance within is to allow yourself to love and be loved.

To cultivate happiness: Walk in beauty, live in trust, and know the benevolent love of God guides your way.

To cultivate internal strength: No one has power over you unless you allow it to happen.

To cultivate truth: Gently and with love, honor yourself.

To cultivate surrender: Gratitude opens the door to feeling God's love.

To cultivate oneness: Be aware of the simple truth that God exists in all circumstances.

• • •

The angelic affirmation system of healing was developed by Shanta Gabriel. If you would like to connect with Shanta, you can reach her at P. O. Box 5275 Kaneohe, Hawaii 96744. Telephone: (808) 239-5433.

Herbal Teas and Tinctures

In ancient times, humankind intuited the knowledge of the herbal kingdom. As the shepherds of ancient times watched their flocks interact with flowers and herbs, they learned which plants had healing affects on the animals. So it was through close and loving observation that cultures in every part of the world developed their own understandings of indigenous plants.

Herbs and flowers provide many medicinal benefits. Teas and tinctures are easy to prepare and use, and can greatly assist in healing of many ailments in a short period of time.

Teas

When preparing herbal teas only use non-metallic containers like glass, earthenware, or enamel. Non-reactive stainless steel can be used as an alternative. Purified water is most preferable, or if it is not available, use distilled water. Avoid tap water because of all its impurities.

There are two different ways to prepare teas. An *infusion* is made from the flowers or soft leaves of the herb or plant. Bring purified water to a boil, take it off the heat, and add the flowers or soft leaves. Cover the container tightly and steep for about twenty minutes, then strain the tea into a clean container.

A *decoction* extracts the deep essences of roots, bark, stems, and stronger leaves. Bring purified water to a boil in an open container and add the herbs. Simmer the herbs, uncovered, for about one hour. About half the water will be lost to evaporation. Strain the tea into a clean container.

Certain herbal formulas combine the use of soft flowers and sturdier barks. To prepare this type of tea, make the decoction first, then pour the strained decoction over the flowers or soft leaves and steep

113

Chapter
Four:
Self
Help
for the
Chakras

for twenty minutes in a tightly sealed container, then strain and store in a clean container.

When preparing an herbal tea for medicinal use, you will use about one ounce of dried herbs to one pint of purified water. When using fresh herbs, double the amount of water.

Tinctures

A tincture is an herbal concentrate in a base of alcohol. Tinctures are easy to take and can be used over long periods of time. Tinctures will last indefinitely because the alcohol base acts as a preservative while fresh herbal teas will only last about three or four days.

To prepare a tincture, sterilize a glass jar and lid in boiling water. On the day of the new moon, combine all of the herbs and alcohol together, and seal the jar tightly. The ratio of herbs to alcohol is four ounces of dried or fresh herbs to one pint of alcohol. The alcohol can be brandy, rum, or vodka. Store the jar in a dark, cool place and shake the jar once a day for fourteen days. On the day of the full moon, strain off the liquid through a cheesecloth or another filter into a sterilized container. The tincture is harvested on the full moon because the waxing moon helps the alcohol extract the healing properties of the herbs.

If you are alcohol-sensitive or do not wish to consume alcohol, remove the lid from the jar of the tincture and place the jar in a pot of water about one and one-half inches deep. Heat the water to about 1200F for about twenty minutes. The alcohol will evaporate. Once the alcohol is removed from the tincture, it will be necessary to refrigerate the tincture for preservation.

Dosage

The typical dosage of medicinal herbal teas in acute situations is one-half cup of tea, taken three times a day. Most acute symptoms can be treated within one week. If the symptoms are chronic and many weeks of treatment are recommended, a tincture of the herbs would be easier to use.

Tinctures are taken in drops. The number of drops will vary according to the strength and type of herbs in the tincture. The stronger the herbs, the fewer number of drops per dosage. Take five to forty drops of the tincture for acute symptoms, three times a day for one week.

If the symptoms are chronic, after two weeks stop the tincture for a few days, then resume the treatment for another two weeks. The body adjusts to the effects of the herbs when they are ingested day after day, and tinctures will then lose their effectiveness. When you stop taking the herbs for a few days, the body has an opportunity to rest. When treatment is resumed, the herbs work at full power again. When using tinctures as a tonic, take fifteen to twenty drops, twice a week. Children usually take half the adult dosage.

Herbal combination to balance the first chakra and the large intestine: Old yam, cardamom, peppermint, marshmallow, and yellow dock.

Herbal combination to balance the second chakra and the reproductive system: Echinacea, cornsilk, horsetail, and parsley root.

Herbal combination to balance the third chakra and the digestive system: Marshmallow, fennel, gentian, and agrimony.

Herbal combination to balance the fourth chakra and the heart and lungs: Hawthorn berry, motherwort, sassafras, mullein, and ginger.

Herbal combinations to balance the fifth chakra and the nervous system: Valerian, nettles, chamomile, and roses.

Herbal combinations to balance the sixth chakra and mental energy: Ginkgo, gota-kola, black cherry, and rosemary.

Herbal combination to balance the seventh chakra and spiritual energy: Mugwort, lavender, skullcap, and damiana.

. . .

There are thousands of herbs to choose from. I have listed just a few combinations. If you study the use of herbs, you will find other herbal

115

Chapter
Four:
Self
Help
for the
Chakras

combinations balance the chakras. It is up to you to experiment and find the herbal combinations that best serve your healing process.

The following are herbal home remedies for some common ailments and complaints:

Burdock and dandelion root tea are excellent blood purifiers.

Celery juice is good for circulation.

Black pepper is good for a cold or flu.

Fennel tea is good for producing mother's milk.

Lemon juice in an eye-wash (one part lemon juice to seven parts water) treats glaucoma or cataracts. To remove gall-stones, drink four ounces of organic, first cold-pressed, extra virgin olive oil with two ounces of fresh-squeezed organic lemon juice

Rosemary, thyme, sage, and clove in a tea treat any foot infection. Use the tea in a bath.

Cabbage, celery, carrot, and lemon: mix juices of these plants with cayenne pepper and drink twice a day to help an ulcer.

Stinging nettle tea in a foot bath helps arthritis.

Orange leaves tea in a bath treat morning sickness.

Cayenne pepper sprinkled in shoes will keep you warm and improve circulation.

Juniper berry tea is good for cramps. Drink daily for one week.

Parsley tea is good for kidney difficulties.

Coffee and parsley are diuretics; stimulating the kidneys.

Garlic soup is good for intestinal worms. Garlic can soften hardening of the arteries, capillaries, and veins. For any ear infection, dip a cotton ball in garlic and olive oil and place the cotton ball in the ear. For a cold or flu, eat two cloves of raw garlic.

Chamomile tea in a warm bath soothes low back pain.

Mugwort tea in a warm bath treats any skin rash.

Raw apple mashed with a little cinnamon will stop diarrhea. For dysentery, add blackberry juice to the apple and cinnamon.

Aloe vera leaf juice is good for digestion. If you are internally hot, drink aloe vera juice for cooling. Aloe vera applied to burns will soothe and heal the skin.

Pranayama

Life cannot exist without the breath. Humans can survive without food for a long period of time, and without water for a shorter period of time, but without the breath, we can only survive for a few short moments. A newborn baby takes in a long deep breath, and as it exhales, its life on Earth begins. Likewise, when it is time to die, we take one last gasp for air before death occurs. From the first breath to the last breath, to breathe is to live.

When breathing, the body takes in air and oxygen and something else called *prana*. Prana is a Sanskrit word describing the life force energy of the universe. Breathing exercises called *pranayama* extract prana from the air.

Prana is not air, but rather the life energy that is part of the air. Prana is everywhere and in all things. Without prana, life would not exist. When we lived in harmony with nature, extracting the prana from the air into the body during respiration was simple. However, twenty-first-century men and women have lost the art of natural breathing. This loss of prana results in the manifestation of diseases. People have lost their connection to nature and replaced it with attachments to the pleasures of the physical world. When we attach to the physical world we hold onto stress and fear. By reconnecting with nature, the stress and fear of worldly living dissipate and the peace presents itself once again. Reconnecting with prana becomes easy.

Pranayama requires breathing through the nostrils. The nostrils act as filters for the respiratory organs. They contain tiny little hairs that catch most of the germs and dust particles that enter the body during inhalation. There are also mucous membranes in the nostrils that warm the air as it passes over them. The lungs can then easily disperse

117

Chapter
Four:
Self
Help
for the
Chakras

the oxygen, and prana to the rest of the body. Mouth breathing has been associated with many physical imbalances. When breathing through the mouth, the air goes directly into the throat and lungs without any dust or germ-catching protection. There are not enough mucous membranes in the throat to sufficiently warm the air. Both the throat and lungs are bombarded with impurities. The impurities from the lungs are passed into the blood as the blood passes through the lungs from the heart to pick up fresh oxygen for distribution to the rest of the body. The end result is sickness and disease for the body.

For best results, practice pranayama in a clean, dry place. Practice pranayama in solitude, in the early morning, or in the evening. Do not eat before practicing pranayama. If you feel tired, do not practice pranayama. Do not bathe after you practice pranayama.

The Whole Breath

The whole breath is a natural breath that gives the body maximum benefit. It is simple, easy to do, and you will notice the benefits immediately. With a little practice, you can incorporate this style of breathing into you life, and be in harmony with nature and the universal life force energy.

All inhalations and exhalations are done through the nostrils. Sit in a chair, or on the floor, or lie down in the corpse position (a yoga pose) on your back, with palms facing up, and your legs and feet a comfortable distance apart. Make sure you are as relaxed as possible and your spine is straight.

Breathe easily in your natural state for ten breaths. Notice how you are breathing. Is your abdominal center involved? How much of your rib cage is involved? Are you breathing shallow or deeply? Just observe your breathing pattern.

On your next breath, as you begin the inhalation, extend your abdominal center outward. Then bring your breath up into your lower rib cage, middle rib cage, upper rib cage and shoulders. As the breath slowly moves upward, let it be one continuous movement. This may take some practice.

Now, slowly exhale in one continuous movement. Repeat this breathing process ten times, slowly increasing to twenty-five times.

The whole breath will relax you, balance your nervous system, and greatly reduce your stress level. For best results, practice at least twice a day.

The following pranayama exercises are designed to help balance the chakras. They are safe and easy to do.

Pranayama to balance the first chakra.

Sit in a chair or cross-legged on the floor. Inhale through both nostrils, slowly and easily. As you inhale, gently tighten the sphincter muscle. Exhale slowly through both nostrils and release the sphincter muscle. Repeat ten times. This will balance the first chakra, and improve the function of the large intestine and lungs.

Pranayama to balance the second chakra.

Sit in a chair or cross-legged on the floor. Inhale through both nostrils in a steady, slow manner. As you exhale through your nostrils, bring your awareness to your sex glands. As you inhale, draw the energy into your sex glands and pull it back to your sacrum. Hold your breath as long as it is comfortable, without straining your back or pelvic muscles. Exhale slowly and repeat ten times. This will balance the second chakra, and improve function of the reproductive system in both men and women.

Pranayama to balance the third chakra.

Sit in a chair or cross-legged on the floor. Inhale through both nostrils, slowly and easily. Exhale slowly through the mouth until all the air is exhaled. Repeat ten times. This will balance the third chakra and improve function of the liver and stomach.

Pranayama to balance the fourth chakra.

Lie down on the floor in the corpse position. Keep your heels together and your hands by your side. Be comfortable and relaxed. With a slow inhalation, raise your hands over your head until they meet the floor above your head. As you exhale, bring your hands back to the sides of your body. Repeat five times. Now, with your hands at your sides, as you

119

Chapter
Four:
Self
Help
for the
Chakras

inhale, raise up your right leg so the sole of your foot is facing the ceiling. As you exhale, slowly bring the right leg down to the floor. Repeat this process with the left leg. Repeat five times with both legs. This will balance the fourth chakra and improve function of the heart and lungs.

Pranayama to balance the fifth chakra.

Sit in a chair or cross-legged on the floor. Inhale through both nostrils. As you exhale through your mouth, pucker your lips and release the breath intermittently until all the air is exhaled. Repeat this breath ten times. This will balance the fifth chakra and improve function to the throat, mouth and face.

Pranayama to balance the sixth chakra.

Lie down in a corpse position. Place both hands over the abdominal center with your fingers interlocked. Inhale into your abdominal center. As you inhale, visualize your abdominal center filling up with the universal life force energy. Now, as you exhale, visualize the universal life force energy from your abdominal center spreading to every part of your body. As the universal life force energy is carried throughout your body, visualize every germ, impurity, diseased tissue or organ, and negative vibrational pattern becoming whole and one with spirit. Repeat twenty times. This will balance the sixth chakra and improve function to the entire body and mind.

Pranayama to balance the seventh chakra.

Sit in a chair or cross-legged on the floor. Inhale easily through both nostrils. After the inhalation is complete, with your right thumb, close off the right nostril, and exhale slowly through your left nostril. When the exhalation is complete, inhale through your left nostril and with your right ring finger, close off the left nostril and exhale slowly through your right nostril. This makes one round. Repeat for ten rounds. This will balance the seventh chakra, reduce stress, balance the nervous system and bring a sense of peace.

There are many pranayama techniques to balance the body, mind, and spirit. It is an exact science perfected by the yogis and saints of India many thousands of years ago. There are pranayama techniques to balance and cure every disease and imbalance known to humankind. I have mentioned just a few.

Yoga Asanas and Energy Mudras

Yoga *asanas* were developed by the yogis and saints of India to assist the body in maintaining its homeostasis. Asanas are stretches and postures that make the nerves and muscles stronger, keep the spine flexible, balance the internal organs, and connect the individual directly with spirit. Two kinds of asanas were developed. The first series of asanas was designed to preserve the body, and keep it free of disease. The second series of asanas was designed to keep the individual comfortable in sitting positions so he could meditate for long periods of time and connect with spirit.

• • •

The following asanas focus on preserving the physical balance of the body, and protect the body against disease.

Asana to balance the first chakra.

Knee to chest. Lie flat on your back with legs stretched out, heels together, and arms extended at your sides. As you inhale through the nostrils, bend your right leg and clasp both hands around your right knee, interlocking your fingers. Pull the knee up to the chest, and lift your head so your nose touches your knee. Hold for a few seconds, then exhale and release the posture. Repeat on the other side. This will complete one round. Practice for five rounds. This asana will also bring relief from constipation, diarrhea, piles, and reduce excess fat from the waist.

121

Chapter
Four:
Self
Help
for the
Chakras

Asana to balance the second chakra.

Head to knee. Sit in a cross-legged position. Straighten out your left leg in front of you, and place your right foot at your left inner thigh. Extend your arms over your head, take a deep breath through your nostrils, and while exhaling slowly, bend forward so your hands reach your toes and your head reaches your knees. Hold for ten seconds. Release the position and reverse on the other side. This will complete one round. Practice for three rounds. This position might seem difficult at first. Most people can not bring their heads to their knees or hands to their toes. Just do the best you can, and with practice you will improve. This asana will also improve flexibility of the low back, hamstring muscles on the back of the legs, create more room in the pelvis, and tonify the reproductive system.

Asana to balance the third chakra.

Bow position. Lie face down with your chin or forehead on the floor. Place your arms by your sides. Bend your legs at your knees, and grasp your feet or ankles with your hands. While inhaling through your nose, lift your head up back; at the same time pull your feet up toward your body with your hands. Hold for five seconds, exhale and release the position. Repeat two times. This will also improve the flexibility of the entire spine, strengthen the stomach, liver, small intestine, and reduce excess fat from the waist.

Asana to balance the fourth chakra.

Camel pose. Sit on your knees with your feet underneath your torso. Keep your spine straight and your arms down by your sides. Inhale through your nostrils, bring your hands back to hold on to your ankles, while dropping your head back and extending your chest forward. While in this position, arch your back, bringing the shoulder blades back close to each other, and stretch your throat as your head drops backward. Hold for a few seconds while continuing to breathe; then release. Repeat two times. This will also improve flexibility of the entire spine, strengthen the heart and lungs, and improve the function of the thyroid gland.

123

Chapter
Four:
Self
Help
for the
Chakras

Asana to balance the fifth chakra.

Fish pose. Lie on your back with your legs stretched out, and your hands by your sides. Slowly arch your back, come up on your elbows, and bring your top of your head to the floor. Hold for five seconds, then release. Repeat two times. This will also improve flexibility to the spine at the low back and neck, strengthen the throat, and improve function of the thyroid gland.

Asana to balance the sixth chakra.

Surrender pose. Lie on your back with your arms at your sides. Bend both legs and bring your feet together so the soles of your feet are facing, but not touching, each other. Your hands come up on to your thighs. Hold for one minute, and gradually increase to ten minutes. This will balance the sixth chakra, and quiet the mind. This is a good position for meditation.

Asana to balance the seventh chakra.

Corpse pose. Lie on your back with your legs stretched out, and the hands by your sides. Be comfortable. Beginning with your feet, and slowly working up your entire body to your head, relax each body part along the way. One by one: feet, ankles, calves, knees, thighs, hips, low back, mid-back, upper-back, shoulders, neck, the length of your arms and hands, and head. Relax your mind by not paying attention to any of your thoughts. Slowly, all thoughts will disappear. This will bring deep relaxation. Stay in the corpse position for fifteen minutes. This will balance the seventh chakra, reduce stress, alleviate fatigue, calm the nervous system, and prepare the individual for meditation.

• • •

While these asanas can be practiced by everyone, women should avoid these poses during their menstrual periods.

Mudras

Energy mudras are derivatives of asanas and are designed to strengthen and balance the endocrine system. The endocrine glands secrete hormones directly into the bloodstream, which carries them to other parts of the body where they regulate the functions of various organs and keep the body healthy and disease-free. The endocrine glands are located at the chakras, and the yoga mudras balance the endocrine glands.

The male endocrine glands, located at the first chakra, are the testes. The testes, located in the lower part of the pelvis, regulate the male reproductive system.

The endocrine glands located at the second chakra are the adrenal glands, and ovaries. The adrenal glands are located on top of the kidneys and regulate a fight or flight response. The ovaries located in the pelvis, regulate the female reproductive system.

The endocrine gland located at the third chakra is the pancreas. The pancreas, located in the abdominal center, regulates digestion.

The endocrine gland located at the fourth chakra is the thymus. The thymus, located in the chest (behind the top part of the breastbone, or sternum), regulates the immune system.

The endocrine gland located at the fifth chakra is the thyroid. The thyroid, located in the throat, regulates metabolism.

The endocrine gland located at the sixth chakra is the pituitary. The pituitary, located just beneath the pineal gland in the center of the brain, is considered to be the master gland because it regulates all the other glands.

The endocrine gland located at the seventh chakra is the pineal. The pineal, located in the middle of the brain, regulates the body's ability to receive and assimilate light.

Yoga mudra to balance the first chakra.

Invigorating mudra. Lie flat on your back with your hands by your sides and your legs straight. Slowly raise your legs upward, and bring your hands to your hips. Hold this position for a few seconds, then release your legs down to the floor. You can increase the amount of time you hold your legs to three to five minutes. This mudra will balance the first chakra, and relieve constipation, and purify the blood.

Yoga mudra to balance the second chakra.

Reproductive mudra. Sit in a straight-back chair or cross-legged on the floor. Inhale slowly and draw the energy up from the coccyx to the reproductive organs, and hold for a few seconds. Exhale and release. Repeat five times. This mudra will balance the second chakra, and tonify the reproductive system in both men and women. This helps move sexual energy up to the brain, and prevents stagnation of energy in the reproductive system.

Yoga mudra to balance the third chakra

Digestive mudra. Stand up with your legs about two and a half feet apart. Place your hands above the knees as you bend forward slightly. Inhale slowly through both nostrils and contract the abdominal muscles toward the spine. Hold the breath for five seconds. Exhale and release. Repeat five times. This mudra will balance the third chakra and invigorate the digestive organs.

Yoga mudra to balance the fourth chakra.

Chest mudra. Sit in a crossed-legged position on the floor. Keep your hands to the sides. Inhale slowly and attempt to bend forward until your forehead touches the floor in front of you. If your forehead does not reach the floor, just do the best you can. Hold for ten seconds. Release and repeat three times. This mudra will balance the fourth chakra, relax the diaphragm, energize the heart and lungs, and create more room in the chest cavity.

Yoga mudra to balance the fifth chakra.

Throat mudra. Sit in a straight-back chair or cross-legged on the floor. Inhale through both nostrils. Exhale slowly and bring the chin down to the breastbone. Hold for a few seconds, then bring the head up and back until the chin is pointing toward the ceiling. Hold for a few seconds. Release and come back to center. Repeat three times. This mudra will balance the fifth chakra, tonify the thyroid gland, and improve communication skills.

125

Chapter
Four:
Self
Help
for the
Chakras

Yoga mudra to balance the sixth chakra.

Brain mudra. Sit in a straight-back chair or cross-legged on the floor. Relax and breathe until you find a comfortable rhythm. Place your left hand across your forehead, and your right hand at the back of your neck. Hold for one to two minutes, then release. This mudra will balance the sixth chakra, energize the brain, and harmonize the pituitary gland.

Yoga mudra to balance the seventh chakra.

Crown mudra. Sit in a straight-back chair or cross-legged on the floor. Relax and breathe until you find a comfortable rhythm. Place your left hand above the top of your head, and your right hand by your coccyx, in the aura. Hold for two minutes. This mudra will balance the seventh chakra and pineal gland, and tonify the entire chakra system.

• • •

These mudras should not be practiced by children under twelve years old. The mudras can activate the sex glands, thyroid gland, and pituitary gland before the natural maturing process. If this occurs, it could hamper a child's normal development of his body, mind and spirit.

Flower Essences

Humankind's special connection with botanicals has developed into symbols of expressions, feelings, and affections. Plants are extremely sensitive, and may act as barometers for measuring people's emotions. The energy fields that radiate from plants can alleviate the toxic, nutritionally deficient, and stress-dominated energy systems of people. The roots of the plant affect the individual's deepest organs, the leaves cleanse the blood, and the flowers are used to restore mental clarity and to reconnect people to spirit.

Flower essences are the extracted subtle energy of flowers in a base of water and alcohol. Flower essences are prepared by gathering certain flowers, putting them in a bowl of purified water, and setting them out to sit in the sun light for about twelve hours. The flowers are strained out of the water, and the water becomes the flower essence. A small amount of alcohol is then added to the water as a preservative. Flower essences have been used to communicate the grace of Mother Nature throughout every culture and civilization. Flower essences communicate their secrets through their cooling and detoxifying nature. Flower essences cool and calm the emotions, resulting in mental clarity. Flower essences affect all of the senses, harmonizing the conscious and subconscious minds.

Flowers only express love. They bloom year 'round to remind us that spirit embraces us in eternal peace, and all our treasures are in our heart.

The Pendulum

People have been using pendulums for thousands of years. The pendulum is a tool for connecting with universal love energy. Used correctly, it determines the highest truth about complex situations, and can answer difficult questions. A pendulum is a heavy object attached to a string or chain about ten inches long. It could be any object, as long as it will dangle when movement is initiated. By asking the pendulum different questions, you can access the truth by the way the pendulum responds.

Periodically, a pendulum must be cleansed to assure its purity (sometimes the pendulum will pick up unwanted energy, which effects its capacity to respond in a truthful manner). To assure that the pendulum is responding to the highest truth from the universe, cleanse it by: burying it in the ground overnight and washing it clean the next morning; let it soak in salt water overnight and wash it clean the next morning; or let cool water run over it for thirty seconds.

To use a pendulum, begin by programming it. Initiate the movement and let the pendulum swing back and forth in front of you. While the pendulum is moving, ask it to show you the way it wants to move to indicate a positive response to a question. The pendulum will either move clock-wise or counterclockwise. Make a note of its response.

Allow the pendulum to swing back and forth again, and ask it to show you the way it wants to move to indicate a negative response. This response should be the opposite of the positive response; however, if it is the same response as the positive one, begin again and use a different object as a pendulum.

The pendulum responds in a neutral way by moving back and forth (not moving clockwise or counterclockwise).

127

Chapter
Four:
Self
Help
for the
Chakras

If you are asking the pendulum to give you an answer about something specific, such as the appropriateness of a remedy or herb or anything that can be held in your hand, place the object in your left hand. With your right hand move the pendulum over the item in question, and ask the pendulum if the item will assist you with your healing process.

If you are asking the pendulum about a situation in your life and there are no objects to be held in your hand, let the pendulum move in front of you, without any objects underneath it. When asking the pendulum about specific, personal issues, the pendulum does not always respond in a clear, truthful manner. This occurs because it is difficult for the individual to channel the truth about his own personal issues. In this situation, ask someone else to use the pendulum to answer the questions about your personal life.

When you are attempting to determine which flower essences should be used to balance a specific complaint or ailment, use a pendulum to determine:

- What flower essence should be used?
- How many days do you need the take the flower essence?
- How often do you need to take the flower essence?
- How many drops from the master bottle (the master bottle is the bottle that the flower essence is packaged in) is considered to be the correct dosage for that individual?
- How many different flower essences can be taken at the same time?

If you are not confident in using a pendulum, the typical dosage is two drops per dose, taken once upon rising and once at bedtime. If you are in an emotional crisis, take the remedies as many times a day as you feel you need to.

There are many different types of flower essences to choose from. I have been using two types of flower essences for many years with wonderful results. The first type is called Petite Fleur Essence, produced by master herbalist Judy Griffin. The second type of flower essence is called Master Flower Essences, produced from the writings and teachings of Paramanhansa Yogananda. The following remedies from Petite Fleur Essences and Master Flower Essences balance the chakras.

Flower essences to balance the first chakra.
Petite Fleur Essences: Zinnia eliminates or decreases the need to be critical of oneself and others.
Master Flower Essences: Fig will soften the need for strict discipline. It helps to break through a self-imposed sense of limitation which allows for greater flexibility of will and spirit.

Flower essences to balance the second chakra.
Petite Fleur Essences: Lilac enables the personality to release past grudges, and promote the self-love that is brought about by forgiveness.
Master Flower Essences: Almond enhances sexual self-control and calms the mind and nerves. It makes it easier to redirect sexual energy and promote inner stillness.

Flower essences to balance the third chakra.
Petite Fleur Essences: Morning Glory allows resistance to change to be replaced by progressive thoughts of faith in oneself. Circulation of the blood increases, opening all physical channels for elimination and purification.
Master Flower Essences: Corn enhances mental vitality. It helps to dispel an attitude of limitation, and brings about the energy for new beginnings. You will acquire more enthusiasm, zeal, and increased energy.

Flower essences to balance the fourth chakra.
Petite Fleur Essences: Garden Mum replaces critical thoughts with a feeling of love for all of beings.
Master Flower Essences: Grape brings about divine love and devotion. It helps uncover the heart's natural ability to love. It awakens the desire to love unconditionally, without the thought of self.

Flower essences to balance the fifth chakra.
Petite Fleur Essences: African Violet touches a cord within spirit to release nurturing and love energy from the soul. This love energy is released into our beings and transforms all negative thoughts and emotions.

129

Chapter
Four:
Self
Help
for the
Chakras

Master Flower Essences: Apple helps to align the physical, mental, and spiritual aspects of the self with the higher self. It helps to channel joy and love; banishing fear, unwillingness, and doubt.

Flower essences to balance the sixth chakra.
Petite Fleur Essences: Azalea enhances personal power of the sixth chakra through wisdom and understanding. It balances all the chakras and encourages the creative energy to flow and flow.
Master Flower Essences: Avocado enhances memory. It helps to keep one mindful of life's goals. It also develops the individual's ability to recognize truth through worldly illusions.

Flower essences to balance the seventh chakra.
Petite Fleur Essences: Sunflower opens the individual to the creator within, allowing the personality to make peace with god.
Master Flower Essences: Orange helps to banish melancholia, and to stimulate the brain. It activates an upward flow of energy to the crown, and helps bring god-awareness to the individual. It also dispels negative moods, depression, and discouragement.

• • •

The following flower essence remedies uplift your spirits and enhance your personal growth:

To cultivate calmness and mental clarity from which creativity can blossom:
Petite Fleur Essences: Iris.
Master Flower Essences: Lettuce.

To cultivate positive thoughts and release doubt and negativity:
Petite Fleur Essences: Red Rose.
Master Flower Essences: Blackberry.

To cultivate calmness and peace within:
Petite Fleur Essences: Sunflower.
Master Flower Essences: Banana.

To cultivate kind-heartedness and recognition of all people as part of the same family:
Petite Fleur Essences: Wisteria.
Master Flower Essences: Raspberry.

To cultivate faith and divine protection:
Petite Fleur Essences: Begonia.
Master Flower Essences: Tomato.

To cultivate joy, wholeness, and groundedness:
Petite Fleur Essences: Daffodil.
Master Flower Essences: Pineapple.

To cultivate dignity and self-worth:
Petite Fleur Essences: Chamomile.
Master Flower Essences: Strawberry.

To cultivate tenderness, sweetness, and remove critical thoughts toward humankind:
Petite Fleur Essences: Garden Mum.
Master Flower Essences: Date.

To cultivate more energy and overcome lethargy:
Petite Fleur Essences: Tiger's Jaw Cactus.
Master Flower Essences: Coconut.

To cultivate peacefulness, relaxation, and meditation:
Petite Fleur Essences: Verbena.
Master Flower Essences: Pear.

• • •

To purchase the Petite Fleur Essence Flower Essences contact Judy Griffin, P.O. Box 330411, Forth Worth, Texas 76163. Telephone: (817) 293-5410. www.aromahealthtexas.com

To purchase the Master Flower Essences contact: Master Flower Essences, 14618 Tyler Road, Nevada City, California 95959. Telephone: (530) 478-7655.

Bija Mantras

Each chakra has a primal sound, called a *bija* mantra. Bija is a Sanskrit word meaning seed or core. Repeating the bija mantras of the chakras purifies the vibrational patterns of the chakras. As the purification process occurs, the chakras either spin off any accumulated excess energy or increase their energy levels if their energy levels are low. The chakras then operate to their maximum potential, ready to receive stimuli from the environment and the universe and respond consciously. A conscious response from the chakra system lets an individual make choices that best serve himself and humankind. All negative thoughts, emotions, and karma can be released, resulting in a complete transformation of the individual. A person can connect to spirit and merge with the universal love energy. Liberation, self-realization, and god-realization can occur.

While working with the bija mantras, it is extremely important to establish a relationship with the mantras. To develop this relationship, one must sit, chant, and meditate with each bija mantra. Chanting a bija mantra at least one hundred and eight times a day for thirty days will establish the desired relationship. The more repetitions of a bija mantra that are chanted on a daily basis, the more quickly an individual's karma will be cleared so the individual can merge with universal love energy. One can also chant more than one bija mantra per day, depending upon the time available.

Often, the number one hundred and eight is associated with chanting or some kind of spiritual discipline. The number one hundred is a complete number and represents God. The remaining number eight represents the eight types of maya of the physical world. They are earth, water, fire, air, space, mind, intellect, and ego. The eight mayas are all that separate humankind from merging completely with spirit.

After a relationship with the bija mantras has been established, an individual will have the ability to immediately clear the chakra system by chanting the bija mantras.

Bija mantra to balance the first chakra.

The bija mantra of the first chakra is *Lam*. It is pronounced with a drawn-out vowel, "Laaaam."

Sit in a straight-back chair or cross-legged on the floor. Inhale slowly through both nostrils, and focus at the coccyx. Connect with the Earth. Feel the Earth. Become one with the Planet Earth. Exhale slowly.

Chant the bija mantra, Lam, one hundred and eight times. As you are chanting Lam, feel the first chakra, and notice how the mantra is affecting this chakra. Each individual can have a different experience, so just become aware of what is happening to you. This technique can be used to balance the energy of the first chakra anytime you feel uncentered, ungrounded, or stuck.

Bija mantra to balance the second chakra.

The bija mantra of the second chakra is *Vam*. It is pronounced with a drawn-out vowel, "Vaaaam."

Sit in a straight-back chair or cross-legged on the floor. Inhale slowly through both nostrils, and focus at the sacrum and pelvis. Connect with the waters of the Earth, and feel the water flowing throughout your body. Exhale slowly.

Chant the bija mantra, Vam, one hundred and eight times. As you are chanting Vam, notice how the sacrum and pelvis feel. This technique can be used to balance the energy of the second chakra anytime you feel spaced out, have low energy, are experiencing an emotional crisis, or need to connect with creative energy.

Bija mantra to balance the third chakra.

The bija mantra of the third chakra is *Ram*. It is pronounced with a drawn-out vowel, "Raaaam."

Sit in a straight-back chair or cross-legged on the floor. Inhale slowly through both nostrils, and focus at the solar plexus. Connect with the heat of the Earth, and feel the warmth flowing throughout your body. Exhale slowly.

Chant the bija mantra, Ram, one hundred and eight times. As you are chanting Ram, notice how your digestive organs are feeling. This technique can be used to balance the energy of the third chakra anytime you feel angry, upset, fearful, or are experiencing digestive difficulties.

133

Chapter
Four:
Self
Help
for the
Chakras

Bija mantra to balance the fourth chakra.

The bija mantra of the fourth chakra is *Yam*. It is pronounced with a drawn-out vowel, "Yaaam."

Sit in a straight-back chair or cross-legged on the floor. Inhale slowly through both nostrils, and focus at the chest. Connect with the universal love energy, and feel love energy flowing throughout your body. Exhale slowly.

Chant the bija mantra Yam, one hundred and eight times. As you are chanting Yam, notice how your heart feels. This technique can be used to balance the energy of the fourth chakra anytime you feel unconnected to love energy, sad, or hurt.

Bija mantra to balance the fifth chakra.

The bija mantra of the fifth chakra is *Ham*. It is pronounced with a drawn-out vowel, "Haaam."

Sit in a straight-back chair or cross-legged on the floor. Inhale slowly through both nostrils, and focus at the throat. Connect with the spaciousness of the universe, and feel the space throughout your body. Exhale slowly.

Chant the bija mantra, Ham, one hundred and eight times. As you are chanting Ham, notice how your throat feels. This technique can be used to balance the energy of the fifth chakra anytime you need to find more direction in life, or if you have difficulty communicating with others.

Bija mantra to balance the sixth chakra.

The bija mantra of the sixth chakra is *Om*. It is pronounced with an elongated O and M, like "ooooommmmm."

Sit in a straight-back chair or cross-legged on the floor. Inhale slowly through both nostrils, and focus at the center of the forehead. Connect with your intuition, and feel your intuitive process throughout your body. Exhale slowly.

Chant the bija mantra, Om, one hundred and eight times. As you are chanting Om, notice how your thought patterns are forming. This technique can be used to balance the energy of the sixth chakra anytime you are feeling mentally unclear or depressed.

Bija mantra to balance the seventh chakra.

The bija mantra of the seventh chakra is *Aum*. It is pronounced with an elongated A and U and M, "aaaaauuuuummmmm."

Sit in a straight-back chair or cross-legged on the floor. Inhale slowly through both nostrils, and focus at the top of the head. Connect with the universal light, and feel peace and bliss throughout your body. Exhale slowly.

Chant the bija mantra, Aum, one hundred and eight times. As you are chanting Aum, notice how you are connected to spirit. This technique can be used to balance the energy of the seventh chakra anytime you are feeling unconnected to spirit, depressed, or lost.

Aromatherapy

Aromatherapy is the use of essential oils extracted from flowers, plants, or herbs, to bring about energetic changes in the body, mind and spirit. These energetic changes release blocked spiritual, mental, emotional, and physical energy, so a person can make new choices that better support herself.

Plants communicate with humankind in many ways. By taking the time to watch, smell, hold, cherish, and sit with plants, the plants enter into your consciousness. The fragrance of plants can intoxicate the senses, bringing peace and tranquility. There is a place in India, high up in the Himalayan Mountains called the Valley of the Flowers. It is said that when people enter this valley and begin to walk through it, they become intoxicated from the fragrances and lose all sense of time, and can wander throughout the valley for days.

Aromatherapy has been enjoyed by every culture and civilization. Aromas enhance an individual's natural beauty, sexual attraction, self-expression, and peace of mind. The stimulating or cooling properties of aromatic oils can uplift your attitude, stabilize your emotional being, enhance tranquillity, and connect you to spirit.

Essential oils are highly concentrated distilled plant essences that enhance the physical, emotional, mental, and spiritual beings. Each different oil reveals the plant's uniqueness, and can assist you in transmuting negative energy into positive energy.

Chapter
Four:
Self
Help
for the
Chakras

Essential oils can be mixed with massage oils, bath and skincare products, perfume bases. Only two or three drops of the essential oil are needed. When used directly on the skin, one drop is enough; more is not better with essential oils. Too much oil can cause an intense irritating reaction to the skin. Do not use essential oils directly in the eyes, nasal passages, or mucus membranes.

Essential oils can only be prepared by distillation. They will last for several years if stored in dark glass in a cool, dry place.

Essential oil to balance the first chakra.
Thyme enhances stamina in troubled times. It reduces chronic fatigue and protects against infectious diseases.

Essential oil to balance the second chakra.
Lavender reduces stress, mood swings, nervousness, and irritability.

Essential oil to balance the third chakra.
Peppermint stimulates digestion and detoxifies the body. It relieves stomach cramps and headaches.

Essential oil to balance the fourth chakra.
Rose evokes the feelings of love, faith, and clarity. Rose comforts in times of sorrow, hurt, and sadness.

Essential oil to balance the fifth chakra.
Geranium balances the endocrine system and the entire body. All body systems work in harmony, and the individual feels peaceful. It also balances depression and anxiety.

Essential oil to balance the sixth chakra.
Basil reduces headaches and calms the mind. It opens the highest creative centers of the brain, and activates the individual's intuition.

Essential oil to balance the seventh chakra.
Rosemary is an uplifting nerve tonic that increases mental awareness, good memory, and enhances the connection to spirit.

• • •

The following essential oils uplift your spirits and enhance your personal growth.

Gardenia attracts more love in your life.

Sage relaxes muscles, and relieves sinus congestion.

Vanilla protects you from negative energy.

White Carnation eases a stubborn attitude.

Columbine helps you to become independent.

Orchid helps resolve past mistakes.

Iris clears mental stress.

Lilac assists with forgiveness.

Pansy assists with the loss of a loved one.

African Violet helps you to love yourself.

Bougainvillea cultivates security within.

Lemon Grass helps resolve rejection.

Marigold balances sexual guilt.

Red Carnation helps resolve feelings of unworthiness.

There are many different companies producing essential oils. Before purchasing essential oils, research the company and product line. Use a pendulum to verify that the product line is of the highest integrity and quality.

137

Chapter
Four:
Self
Help
for the
Chakras

Color Healing

Color healing uses the colors of the rainbow to harmonize a person with her physical, mental, emotional, and spiritual energies. Colors affect the spiritual energy of the body and each color of the rainbow is directly associated with a specific chakra.

Every subtle energy system, organ, and chakra of the body vibrates at a certain level. When the vibrational rate of these subtle energies are vibrating with too little or too much energy, imbalances can occur. Bathing the individual in the appropriate color will restore the harmonious vibrational rate. Color healing is completely safe, has no side effects, and can be used to restore health for every type of imbalance and disease.

At one time, the energy of the universe was perfect. It was beyond duality, form, and sound. For some unknown reason, a spontaneous stirring within the depths of space created movement within this perfect energy. The movement created a vibrational shift of the energy, and the energy began to manifest into the physical form of matter. Within the universe, matter created duality, expressed as darkness and light. Darkness corresponds to the feminine energy, and light corresponds to the masculine energy. Colors arose from both the darkness and the light. Colors are part of an individual's core energy, affecting every cell in his body.

All forms of matter, including human beings, contain a part of the original perfect energy of the universe. Colors are part of the original form of matter. Humans have forgotten their spiritual connection to the universal energy because of their attachment to the physical world. When an individual is unconnected to spirit, he suffers and experiences emotional, mental, and physical pain that may manifest as disease. Color healing can be the bridge that reconnects an individual with the perfect energy of the universe. Individuals can heal themselves, the Earth, and the entire Universe by using color therapy.

Red balances the first chakra.

The color red is drawn into the body through the first chakra. It is uplifting and expansive; increases confidence, and invigorates the energy of an individual. It assists in overcoming depression, low energy, fear and worry, improves circulation, and promotes a strong mental state. Red is used to heal people who have weak blood, anemia, and low vitality.

Orange balances the second chakra.

The color orange is drawn into the body through the second chakra. It expands the mind to accept new concepts and thoughts. It uplifts the emotions, especially if one is depressed. It also helps break through old patterns and resistance to change. Orange is used to heal the spleen, kidneys, gall bladder, and lungs.

Yellow balances the third chakra.

The color yellow is drawn into the body through the third chakra. It stimulates the mind and increases mental powers. As the mind clears, the emotions are better controlled. The yellow color helps the individual's attitude become positive, creating a happy mental state. All of the digestive organs receive benefit from the yellow color, and it is especially good for the liver and skin. The yellow color is used to heal skin difficulties, nervousness, indigestion, and diabetes. It is also good for mental exhaustion.

Green balances the fourth chakra.

The green color is drawn into the body through the fourth chakra. It brings a feeling of peace and tranquillity. Green is renewing and rejuvenating, and assists an individual in feeling whole. The heart receives a tremendous benefit from the green color, and all of an individual's irritated emotions are soothed. Green calms, and assists an individual in getting in touch with his softer side. Green is used to heal all conditions of the heart. It balances the nervous system, and harmonizes the entire body.

Blue balances the fifth chakra.

The color blue is drawn into the body through the fifth chakra. It helps an individual calm herself, especially if she has been agitated. An individual becomes peaceful and tranquil; her nervous system is brought into balance. Blue controls an individual's ability to speak and communicate with others. It also helps the body fight infection. Blue is used to heal fevers, throat difficulties, inflammations, insect bites, headaches, stress, and sleep disorders.

Indigo balances the sixth chakra.

The color indigo is drawn into the body through the sixth chakra. It helps individual overcome mental disorders such as psychosis. It opens the psychic pathways, and improves intuitive abilities. Indigo purifies the blood, and helps the mind be free of inhibitions. It balances the nervous system and assists with ear, eye, and nose diffi-

139

Chapter
Four:
Self
Help
for the
Chakras

culties. It helps an individual become aware of his higher self, deepening his understanding of the meaning of life. The indigo color is used to heal the lungs, throat, and asthma.

Violet balances the seventh chakra.
The color violet is drawn into the body through the seventh chakra. It is the best color to assist in gaining awareness of spirit. It connects an individual to the highest spiritual energy, assisting her with knowledge of her intuition. Violet soothes and calms the nervous system, bringing a sense of peace to the individual. The color violet is used to heal all mental disorders. It is also used for any nervous imbalance, for joint difficulties, and kidney problems.

Healing with Colors

Use a pendulum (see page 127) to determine which chakra is out of balance. A practitioner can use his intuition, or listen to her client's symptoms to determine which chakra is out of balance.
Have the client sit in a chair or lie on a massage table.

Use a color lamp (a lamp with interchangeable colored bulbs, or a lamp with interchangeable colored slides) to bathe the client in the appropriate color to balance the symptom or complaint. Usually, the session will last about fifteen minutes.

Let purified water sit in the sunlight in a colored jar or glass for two to four hours. The color of the glass or jar needs to be the appropriate color to heal the symptoms of the client. If the practitioner does not have a colored glass or jar, he can place a colored lid over a regular jar or glass. The client drinks the color-charged water to assist in healing the chakra that is out of balance.

Direct the client to inhale the healing color through his nostrils, and visualize the color going to the chakra that is out of balance. Then, exhale all the impurities and negative energy that has been stored at that chakra. Repeat five times.

Gemstone Healing

Gemstones and minerals are nature's gift to humankind. They have been used for currency, art, and jewelry. Gemstones and minerals carry a certain vibration that has always attracted humankind to touch, admire, collect, and trade them. Humankind's love of gemstones and minerals has evolved in all cultures, religions, races, customs, and societies. Besides being greatly admired for their beauty, gemstones and minerals have also been used to heal people for thousands of years.

Ancient healers recognized that gemstones and minerals had different healing effects upon the human body. Certain stones would soothe and calm, while others would uplift spirits and energize a person. Through intuition and meditation, ancient healers mapped out a system of energy balancing that correlated certain gemstones and minerals to certain chakras. By placing certain gemstones and minerals at different chakras, the ancient healers discovered how to help people heal themselves from many different kinds of imbalances and diseases.

141

Chapter
Four:
Self
Help
for the
Chakras

Gemstones and minerals to balance the first chakra.
Ruby, garnet, smoky quartz, bloodstone.

Gemstones and minerals to balance the second chakra.
Coral, amber, pearl.

Gemstones and minerals to balance the third chakra.
Topaz, amber, citrine, tiger eye, gold.

Gemstones and minerals to balance the fourth chakra.
Green jade, emerald, rose quartz, tourmaline, malachite.

Gemstones and minerals to balance the fifth chakra.
Lapis, turquoise, aquamarine, blue topaz.

Gemstones and minerals to balance the sixth chakra.
Lapis, onyx, quartz, sodalite, selenite, amethyst.

Gemstones and minerals to balance the seventh chakra.
Diamond, quartz, selenite, amethyst, purple fluorite.

Gemstone Healing Technique

Place your client on his back on a massage table, or futon on the floor. Place whatever gemstone or mineral to be used for healing directly over the chakra. The practitioner can use gemstones and minerals for all seven chakras simultaneously, or for one or two chakras at a time, depending the client's needs. More is not necessarily better. After the gemstones and minerals are in place, have the client breathe into the chakra that needs to be balanced. The client can inhale the energy of the gemstone or mineral into the chakra, and exhale out the negative energy of the chakra. This can be repeated up to ten breaths for each chakra.

When done, have the client visualize being surrounded by white light, and let him bathe in the white light for five minutes. This will soothe and balance all his energy.

Balancing
the
Chakras

Chapter Five
Chakra Healing through Meditation

The art of meditation is simple. It is only the restlessness of the human mind that makes it appear difficult. When the mind is quiet and all unnecessary mental activity ceases to disturb an individual's equilibrium, a state of meditation is achieved. Meditation is a state of consciousness in which the mind surrenders its power of control and allows the soul to operate the body. When the soul energy operates the body, an individual connects with her spiritual essence, the Planet Earth, the Solar System, and the Universe. She becomes one with everything. There is no longer any separation between her and the rest of creation. She is in sync with the land, water, fire, air, sound waves, light waves, and any manifestation of energy that exists, on any level.

Meditation is a state of consciousness where all things meet on an energy level. Once an individual achieves a state of energetic union with all aspects of creation, he becomes transcendental, and is forever bonded to the cosmic consciousness. In meditation, all of maya is pierced by the thunderbolt of white light, and a person no longer identifies with the physical world or ego. The consciousness of the individual who meditates seeks to transcend the dualistic concepts that keep humankind bound to birth and death, and rebirth. The individual detaches from people, places, and things and journeys down the road of life free of all bondage from the Earthly plane. Totally immersed in the energy of cosmic consciousness, the individual who meditates is truly free to be.

Many people know the concept of meditation, but few take the time to learn the technique and fewer still practice meditation. It appears that most people are just too busy: too involved with their worldly experiences, spending too much time going here and there, earning money or raising a family to find the time for meditation. It is sad that twenty-first-century human beings have missed opportunities to connect with spirit through meditation. When asked about meditation, people sometimes say, " I'll do it later," or "After I get a million dollars, I'll meditate." People put other things first and don't realize that becoming one with spirit is the purpose of being alive. By becoming attached to worldly things, the individual forgets who he really is, and what his purpose in life is.

Meditation is the bridge from the physical world to the spiritual world. In the physical world, the individual can experience attachment to people, places, and things. There will be pain, suffering, and a longing to be loved. In the spiritual world, the individual can experience peace, joy, happiness, clarity, absolute love, truth, and oneness with all things in the universe. The choice belongs to the individual!

You may use any of the information in the self-help sections to assist in conjunction with the meditation techniques described in this section. Often, it takes a strong commitment of follow-up care to maintain a healthy chakra system. It is recommended that you use some of the self-help techniques to keep you chakras operating in a balanced way. The more time and energy you spend caring for your chakra system, the healthier you will be.

Healing the Chakras
1. Create a meditation space.
2. Create a prayer table.
3. Prepare for meditation.
4. Discover which chakra is out of balance.
5. Use guided meditations to heal the chakras.

1. Create a Meditation Space.
Creating a place to meditate in your home will give you the space to practice meditation and alleviate the burden of not knowing how to begin. Ideally, one would like to have a specific room for the practice of meditation. If you do not have a specific room for meditation, create a meditation space in the most quiet and least-traveled part of

your home. A separate room or quiet space is recommended for this will allow the meditation energy to build up in that area. This is important. Every time you meditate, the energy will get stronger and stronger in the meditation space. This will create a place of peace, tranquillity, and strong spiritual energy. Ultimately, the meditation place will be transformed into a powerful spiritual force within the home. It will help you connect with spirit as soon as you enter the space. If the meditation space is not a quiet place, or many people pass through the meditation area (like a living room), it will dissipate the meditation energy.

It is recommended that you get a special meditation cushion to sit on. The cushion should only be used by you and is not to be shared with others. It should be hand-made of natural fibers, or purchased with the intention of only using it for meditation. If you do not want to use a cushion, a comfortable bench or mat can be substituted.

2. Create a Prayer Table.

The prayer table needs to be big enough to hold a few meditation objects. I have a small wooden prayer table about two feet high, one-and-a-half feet long by one-and-a-half feet wide. It is covered with a clean, cotton cloth (synthetic fabrics block the flow of energy). I have a candle, incense and holder, fresh flowers, prayer beads, special stones, crystals, and a picture of my spiritual teacher on my prayer table. Choose whatever spiritual objects are important to you for your prayer table.

The prayer table will become a source of empowerment. As time goes by, with continuous meditation, spiritual energy will slowly build at the prayer table. It will become a place of peace and tranquillity within your home.

3. Prepare for Meditation.

Before you meditate, be sure that you will not be hurried and have ample time to complete the meditation. If your time is limited, it will be best to reschedule your meditation. You will have best results by setting everything else aside and focusing on yourself while you meditate. All of your other responsibilities and duties should be put on hold.

Establishing a daily meditation routine will bring continued success. Practicing meditation at the same time every day is the easiest way to establish a sense of commitment. Just as your body expects to ingest food at a specific time of the day, your soul will look forward to meditating at a specific time of day. If it is impossible for you to meditate at the same time each day, meditate when it is convenient. The only time meditation is not recommended is after eating a meal; wait approximately three hours. Women should avoid meditation during their menstruation cycle.

Some people will meditate in the morning, some in the afternoon, and some in the evening. Some people will have the discipline to meditate every day, while others will not. However the meditation practice manifests for you, it is okay. No one is perfect, and it will not serve you to become upset with yourself if you have any difficulty in establishing a regular meditation practice. With time, concentration, and determination, you will overcome any obstacle that prevents you from meditating.

It is important to have no expectations about the outcome of meditation. Without any predetermined wants or desires, you will be free to experience the meditation at its deepest level. Sometimes, you will be able to enter into a deep state of meditation quickly and easily. Other times you will not be able to quiet your mind, and meditation will be difficult to achieve. Whatever occurs for you during meditation is exactly what is needed. Not judging the results keep the meditation pure.

Now you are ready to sit with consciousness at the prayer table. Light the candle and incense. Chant the mantra "om" three times. Sit quietly for five minutes, and practice the whole breath (see page 119). This will quiet the mind and balance the nervous system. Set your intention. If you want to meditate to heal a specific imbalance or disease, set your intention for that purpose. Cosmic law states that energy always follows intention. Set the intention and let the energy do the rest. If you do not have any specific plan for this meditation, and just want to meditate for general well being, meditate to have your soul current come into balance. When the soul current comes into balance, it automatically heals all other aspects of you.

4. Discover which chakra is out of balance.

You can discover which chakra is out of balance by using intuition, a pendulum, or by checking with the symptom list in the Appendix.

5. Use guided meditations to heal the chakras.

Choose from the following three guided meditations to heal any of the chakras that might be out of balance.

Rainbow Meditation

The rainbow meditation will relax you, reduce systemic stress, and help you feel one with spirit. This meditation can be used whenever you feel the need to change your energy, regardless of the time of day or situation. This meditation will assist you in attaining gentle, peaceful days.

Lie down on the floor in the corpse position, with palms facing upward, or sit in the full lotus or half-lotus position, in a chair, or cross-legged on the floor. You need to be comfortable in the position you choose.

Begin the meditation by focusing on the breath. Breathe through your nostrils (no mouth breathing) in an easy, rhythmic manner. As you inhale, push your belly out, taking the breath up into your chest. Now, exhale through both nostrils. This will help the diaphragm expand and contract, giving you a complete breath. Continue to breathe this way for twenty breaths. You will become relaxed and quiet from conscious breathing.

Now focus your energy on your mind. At first, just watch the different thoughts pass by. You do not react or respond to any of this ongoing mental energy—just let it be. After a time, your mind will become empty and blank.

Now place your awareness at the first chakra. Imagine the color red in this area. As the red color comes into the coccyx area, notice how you feel. Do you notice any emotions or memories? Whatever occurs is okay. Do not attempt to stop anything from occurring. Keep your focus on the red color, and continue to breathe.

Now place your awareness at the second chakra. Imagine the color orange in this area. As the orange color comes into the sacrum area, notice how you feel. Do you notice any emotions or memories? Whatever occurs is okay. Do not attempt to stop anything from occurring. Keep your focus on the orange color, and continue to breathe.

Now places your awareness at the third chakra. Imagine the color yellow in this area. As the yellow color comes into the navel center and mid-back areas, notice how you feel. Do you notice any emotions or memories? Whatever occurs is okay. Do not attempt to stop anything from occurring. Keep your focus on the yellow color, and continue to breathe.

Now place your awareness at the fourth chakra. Imagine the color green in this area. As the green color comes into the chest and upper back area, notice how you feel. Do you notice any emotions or memories? Whatever occurs is okay. Do not attempt to stop anything from occurring. Keep your focus on the green color, and continue to breathe.

Now place your awareness at the fifth chakra. Imagine the color blue in this area. As the sky blue color comes into the throat and neck, notice how you feel. Do you notice any emotions or memories? Whatever occurs is okay. Do not attempt to stop anything from occurring. Keep your focus on the blue color, and continue to breathe.

Now place your awareness at the sixth chakra. Imagine the color indigo in this area. As the indigo color comes into your forehead and brain, notices how you feel. Do you notice any emotions or memories? Whatever occurs is okay. Do not attempt to stop anything from occurring. Keep your focus on the indigo color, and continue to breathe.

Now place your awareness at the seventh chakra. Imagine the color violet in this area. As the violet color comes into the top of the head, notices how you feel. Do you notice any emotions or memories? Whatever occurs is okay. Do not attempt to stop anything from occurring. Keep your focus on the violet color, and continue to breathe.

Now, you have all the colors of the rainbow in alignment with your central core—red, orange, yellow, green, blue, indigo, and violet. You can be quiet for the next ten minutes, enjoying the rainbow within.

After ten minutes have passed, gently come out of the meditation by slowly moving your hands, fingers, feet, and toes, and, finally the rest of your body. Practice this meditation once a day for one month. This will give you the confidence and ability to focus on any chakra when that chakra needs help.

Chakra Awareness Meditation

The chakra awareness meditation can be used to quiet the entire chakra system or for the specific healing of an individual chakra. This meditation will relax you, bring peace of mind, and connect you to the spiritual energy of your chakra system.

Lie down in the corpse position with palms facing upward. You can also sit cross-legged on the floor. You need to be comfortable in the position you choose. Breathe through your nostrils (no mouth breathing) in an easy, rhythmic manner. As you inhale, push your belly out, taking the breath up into your chest. Now, exhales through both nostrils. This will help the diaphragm expand and contract, giving you a complete breath. Continue to breathe this way for twenty breaths. You will become relaxed and quiet from conscious breathing.

Now focus your energy on your mind. At first, just watch the different thoughts pass by. You do not react or respond to any of this ongoing mental energy—just let it be. After a time, your mind will become empty and blank.

Now, place your awareness at the seventh chakra. Breathe into the chakra. Notice how the chakra feels. Can you feel the entire crown chakra? Does you feel the center of the chakra or its perimeter? Does the chakra feel warm or cool? Does the chakra feel like it is tingling? Can you describe what you feel at you crown chakra? Whatever you experience is okay. Do not attempt to force the energy and make something happen. Just let it be, continue to breathe, and be aware.

When you begin to experience awareness at the crown chakra, you might feel a pulsing or tingling sensation, or the crown chakra might become sensitive to the touch. You might see white light, or rainbow colors in your mind. You might feel a great connection to the universal love energy, or feel love for all things. The experience can be life changing.

Now place your awareness at the sixth chakra. Breathe into the chakra. Notice how the chakra feels. Can you feel the third eye? Do you feel the center of the chakra or its perimeter? Does the chakra feel warm or cool? Does the chakra feel like it is tingling? Can you describe what you feel at your third eye? Whatever you experience is okay. Do not attempt to force the energy and make something happen. Just let it be, continue to breathe, and be aware.

When you begin to experience awareness at the third eye, you might feel a cooling or vibrating sensation. You might feel like the third eye is opening like a flower blooming. You might become aware of situations and events that occurred in past lives, or see events of the future. Your powers of intuition might be increased. You can have a new awareness about things and situations in your life, and figure out new solutions to difficult problems.

Now place your awareness at the fifth chakra. Breathe into the chakra. Notice how the chakra feels. Can you feel the throat chakra? Do you feel the center of the chakra or its perimeter? Does the chakra feel warm or cool? Does the chakra feel like it is tingling? Can you describe what you feel at the throat chakra? Whatever you experience is okay. Do not attempt to force the energy and make something happen. Just let it be, continue to breathe, and be aware.

When you begin to experience awareness at the throat chakra, your perceptions about acceptance begin to change. You become more tolerant and patient in stressful situations. You develop clarity in communication skills, and can easily talk about your inner truth. You begin to walk your talk. You can easily maintain your integrity, and your high code of ethics becomes an example for others.

151

Chapter
Five:
Chakra
Healing
through
Meditation

Now, place your awareness at the fourth chakra. Breathe into the chakra. Notice how the chakra feels. Can you feel the heart chakra? Do you feel the center of the chakra or its perimeter? Does the chakra feel warm or cool? Does the chakra feel like it is tingling? Can you describe what you feel at your heart chakra? Whatever you experience is okay. Do not attempt to force the energy and make something happen. Just let it be, continue to breathe, and be aware.

When you begin to experience awareness at the heart chakra, you feel unconditional love for all beings and things. The love energy just pours out from your chest, expanding to all parts of the universe. Whatever sadness, hurt, or grief you might be holding onto is resolved in an easy way. You are free to love and be loved.

Now place your awareness at the third chakra. Breathe into the chakra. Notice how the chakra feels. Can you feel the entire navel chakra? Do you feel the center of the chakra or its perimeter? Does the chakra feel warm or cool? Does the chakra feel like it is tingling? Can you describe what you feel at your navel chakra? Whatever you experience is okay. Do not attempt to force the energy and make something happen. Just let it be, continue to breathe, and be aware.

When you experience awareness at the solar plexus chakra, suppressed emotions like anger, fear, and hurt can surface. It will present a wonderful opportunity for you to resolve and clear these suppressed emotions. You will then feel lighter and happier. Your digestion will improve. You will be less likely to control others and you will stop attempting to be perfect. You will also have a clearer vision of your goals in life, and your mind will cease being so intense with thoughts.

Now place your awareness at the second chakra. Breathe into the chakra. Notice how the chakra feels. Can you feel the entire sacral chakra? Does you feel the center of the chakra or its perimeter? Does the chakra feel warm or cool? Does the chakra feel like it is tingling? Can you describe what you feel at your sacral chakra? Whatever you experience is okay. Do not attempt to force the energy and make something happen. Just let it be, continue to breathe, and be aware.

When you begin to experience awareness at the second chakra, your creativity flows freely. You can use this creative energy to draw, paint, write, sing, dance, or however else it manifests. You will come into balance with your emotions, and not have the need to go up and down emotionally. Your sexual energy will be in harmony, and you will be able to be intimate on the physical level. Your kidneys and reproductive system will be healed and you will have an endless supply of energy for all of your projects.

Now place your awareness at the first chakra. Breathe into the chakra. Notice how the chakra feels. Can you feel the entire root chakra? Does you feel the center of the chakra or its perimeter? Does the chakra feel warm or cool? Does the chakra feel like it is tingling? Can you describe what you feel at your root chakra? Whatever you experience is okay. Do not attempt to force the energy and make something happen. Just let it be, continue to breathe, and be aware.

When you begin to experience awareness at the first chakra, you feel safe and secure. You are no longer worried about how you are going to survive in the world. You become content with what you have, and are grateful to be alive. You become more flexible in your attitudes and actions, and no longer hold on to past negative emotions. The function of the large intestine is improved, and you feel lighter.

Now your energy is ready to ascend upward along the spine, from the tip of the coccyx to the top of the crown, chakra by chakra. As your energy ascends along the spine, reconnect with each chakra. Your goal is just to feel the energy of each chakra, as the energy moves upward toward the crown. Some of the chakras will feel clear and light, while others might feel heavy or stuck. Do not judge the energy of each chakra; just be aware of the differences in their energies. The more you practice this meditation, the more you will notice the chakras come into balance and the entire chakra system operating in harmony.

Each cycle consists of bringing the awareness of the individual from the crown chakra to the root chakra, then back up to the crown chakra. Beginning at the crown chakra, repeat the process for five cycles. Practice this meditation everyday for one month. It will give you the confidence and ability to focus on any chakra, whenever that chakra needs to be balanced.

Complementary Chakra Meditation

This meditation is designed to reduce stress, bring a new awareness to the chakras, balance the energy flowing within the chakra system, and assist you in finding homeostasis.

Lie down in the corpse position with palms facing upward, or sit cross-legged on the floor. You must be comfortable in the position he chooses. Breathe through your nostrils (no mouth breathing) in an easy, rhythmic manner. As you inhale, push your belly out, taking the breath up into your chest. Now, exhale through both nostrils. This will help the diaphragm expand and contract, giving you a complete breath. Continue to breathe this way for twenty breaths. You will become relaxed and quiet from conscious breathing.

Now focus your energy on your mind. At first, just watch the different thoughts pass by. You do not react or respond to any of this ongoing mental energy—just let it be. After a time, your mind will become empty and blank.

Place your awareness at the seventh chakra. Begin by slowly breathing into the chakra. Notices how the chakra feels. Visualize the color violet coming into the crown chakra. Now place your awareness at the first chakra and notice how the first chakra feels. Visualize the color red coming into the first chakra. Now, you have your focus on both the crown and root chakras, with the red and violet colors increasing your awareness. Notices how it feels to have the top and bottom of your chakra system vibrating simultaneously. There is no judgment. Just observing and feeling the experience.

This connection will strengthen the entire chakra system, and help in healing both chakras. Whenever you determine that either the crown chakra or root chakra is out of balance, bringing your awareness to both of them simultaneously will heal both.

Now place your awareness at the sixth chakra. Begin by slowly breathing into the chakra. Notices how the chakra feels. Visualize the color indigo coming into the third eye. Now place your awareness at the second chakra and notice how it feels. Visualize the color orange coming into the second chakra. Now, your have your focus on both the sixth and second chakras, with the indigo and orange colors increasing your awareness of the chakras. Notice how it feels to have the sixth and second chakras vibrating simultaneously. There is no judgment. You are just observing and feeling the experience.

This connection will assist you in healing both of these chakras. Whenever you determine that either the sixth or second chakra is out of balance, you can bring you awareness to them simultaneously and heal both chakras.

Now place your awareness at the fifth chakra. Begin by slowly breathing into the chakra. Notices how the chakra feels. Visualize the color blue coming into the throat chakra. Now, place your awareness at the third chakra and notice how it feels. Visualize the yellow color coming into the third chakra. Now, you have your focus on both the fifth and third chakras, with the blue and yellow colors increasing your awareness. Notice how it feels to have the fifth and third chakras vibrating simultaneously. There is no judgment. You are just observing and feeling the experience.

This connection will assist you in healing both of these chakras. Whenever you determine that either the fifth or third chakra is out of balance, you can bring his awareness to them simultaneously and heal both chakras.

Now place your awareness at the fourth chakra. Begin by slowly breathing into the chakra. Notices how the chakra feels. Visualizes the color green coming into the chakra. Once the green color is in place at the fourth chakra, allow the green color to expand throughout the rest of your body. Visualizes the green color traveling down to your legs and feet, down your arms and hands, to your neck and head, along your back, and into your pelvis. As the green color permeates your body, your being is filled with love energy. The love energy transmutes any negative energy that you might be holding onto.

This meditation will assist you in healing your entire chakra system. The more you practice this meditation, the easier it becomes.

Appendix One
Symptoms and Imbalances of the Chakras

The following are lists of symptoms and imbalances associated with the seven chakras. Some of the same symptoms will be listed at different chakras. When this occurs, balance both chakras that contain the same symptoms.

Remember to go slow and easy. This is not a race against time. Healing is a process, let the process unfold in a natural way. Be gentle with yourself, and don't attempt to do everything at once. Experiment with the guided meditations and the self-help remedy to determine what works for you.

First Chakra Symptoms and Imbalances

- Addictive-Obsessive Behavior
- Ankle tightness
- Attachment to things and emotional difficulties
- Boils
- Bone difficulties
- Bowel difficulties
- Cancer of the large intestine
- Cataracts
- Coccyx difficulties
- Colon difficulties
- Complaining
- Constipation
- Controlling
- Corns and calluses
- Deafness
- Depression
- Diarrhea
- Feeling unloved
- Dominating personality
- Egotistical
- Fear of survival
- Feeling disoriented
- Feeling lack of support
- Feeling nobody cares
- Feeling not good enough
- Feeling ungrounded
- Feeling unwanted
- Gas pain
- Gout
- Headache
- Hemorrhoids
- Illusions
- Indecisiveness
- Inflexibility
- Insecurity
- Internal tightness
- Irritable bowel syndrome
- Irritation
- Joint difficulties
- Knee difficulties
- Lack of balance
- Laziness
- Lethargy
- Loss of sense of smell
- Lower leg difficulties
- Lower spine difficulties
- Male reproductive difficulties
- Materialism
- Muscular difficulties
- Neckache
- Obesity
- Osteoporosis
- Paralysis
- Physically weak
- Piles
- Polyps
- Prostate difficulties
- Resentfulness
- Rheumatism
- Rigidity
- Snoring
- Stiffness
- Suicidal feelings
- Teeth difficulties
- Throat difficulties
- Tumor
- Uncenteredness
- Warts
- Workaholism

Appendix One: Symptoms and Imbalances of the Chakras

Second Chakra Symptoms and Imbalances

- Abscess
- Acne
- Addictive behavior
- Adrenal disorder
- Alcoholism
- Anemia
- Athlete's foot
- Bedsores
- Bedwetting
- Being a loner
- Bladder difficulties
- Bleeding
- Blood disorders
- Body odor
- Boils
- Breast cancer
- Breast difficulties
- Bruises
- Cancer of the blood
- Canker sore
- Caretaking
- Chlamydia
- Clogged arteries
- Crisis-oriented
- Crying
- Cysts
- Dandruff
- Defensive
- Diverticulitis
- Drug addiction

- Dry skin
- Eczema
- Edema
- Emotional stuffing
- Extreme sensitivity
- Fallen Arches
- Fear
- Feeling withdrawn
- Fever blisters
- Flat feet
- Frigidity
- Gangrene
- Greed
- Guilt
- Hernias
- Herpes
- Hostility,
- Impotency
- Kidney difficulties
- Lack of creativity
- Lack of trust, with-
  drawn
- Loss of taste
- Low back pain
- Lupus
- Lymphatic
  difficulties
- Measles
- Menopause
  difficulties
- Menstruation
  difficulties

- Mononucleosis
- Nose bleed
- Ovarian disorders
- Overly assertive
- Overly emotional
- Passive-aggressive
  behavior
- Periodontal disease
- Physical indulgence
- Premenstrual
  syndrome
- Pridefulness
- Prostate difficulty
- Psoriasis
- Rabies
- Reticence
- Rheumatism
- Sciatica
- Sex addiction
- Sexual frigidness
- Sinus difficulties
- Skin difficulties
- Swollen ankles
- Urinary Tract
  difficulties
- Uterine difficulties
- Vaginitis
- Varicose veins
- Venereal Disease
- Yeast infection

Third Chakra Symptoms and Imbalances

- Abdominal cramps
- Aluminum toxicity
- Anger
- Anorexia
- Appetite difficulties
- Arrogance
- Arsenic poisioning
- Arterial problems
- Ateriosclerosis
- Bad breath
- Bee sting
- Belching
- Blisters
- Body odor
- Boils
- Burns
- Cancers
- Cancer of digestive organs
- Cataracts
- Cellulite
- Chicken pox
- Cholesterol
- Circulatory problems
- Cold hands
- Colic
- Conjunctivitis
- Control issues
- Demanding
- Depression
- Diabetes
- Diaphragm difficulties
- Digestion difficulties
- Dominating
- Easily frustrated
- Excess gas
- Eye problems
- Fatigue
- Fear
- Fever
- Gall bladder
- Glaucoma
- Gout
- Heartburn
- Hepatitis
- Hives
- Hypertension
- Hyperventilation
- Indigestion
- Infections
- Inflammation
- Itching
- Jaundice
- Lack of concentration
- Lack of confidence
- Lead poisoning
- Liver difficulties
- Mental confusion
- Middle back troubles
- Multiple sclerosis
- Myopia
- Nausea
- Not trusting
- Pancreas difficulties
- Perfectionism
- Poison ivy, poison oak
- Power issues
- Rabies
- Rashes
- Rudeness
- Sarcasm
- Small intestine difficulties
- Spleen
- Stomach
- Sunburn
- Ulcers
- Unhappiness
- Vengefulness
- Workaholism
- Worry

Appendix
One:
Symptoms
and
Imbalances
of the
Chakras

Fourth Chakra Symptoms and Imbalances

- Allergies
- Angina
- Anxiety disorder
- Arteriosclerosis
- Asthma
- Bedwetting
- Being abused
- Breast difficulties
- Breathing disorders
- Bronchitis
- Calf pain
- Cannot reach out
- Chest pain
- Chronic pain
- Croup
- Crying
- Deceitful
- Difficulty with arms
- Difficulty with love relationships
- Dullness
- Emphysema
- Fainting

- Fatigue
- Fear of the unknown
- Feeling closed off
- Feeling loveless
- Grief
- Guilt
- Hand problems
- Hay Fever
- Headache
- Heart attack
- Heart difficulties
- Indecisiveness
- Joylessness
- Kidney disease
- Lack of compassion
- Lack of confidence
- Lack of openness
- Lack of respect
- Lack of tenderness
- Lack of understanding
- Lack of warmth
- Lung disorders
- Making ultimatums

- Mononucleosis
- Moodiness
- Nail biting
- Never satisfied
- No boundaries
- Not trusting
- Numbness
- Pneumonia
- Rationalizing and intellectualizing
- Rounded shoulders
- Sadness
- Scapula difficulties
- Shame
- Skin disorders
- Smoking
- Thymus difficulties
- Tight shoulders
- Trapezius difficulties
- Unforgiving
- Upper back troubles
- Victim role
- Will not ask for help

Fifth Chakra Symptoms and Imbalances

- Accidents
- Aches
- Amnesia
- Anxiety
- Any change in speech
- Arteriosclerosis
- Arthritis
- Burnout
- Bursitis
- Carpal tunnel syndrome
- Chronic disease
- Colds
- Communication difficulties
- Compulsive behavior
- Controlling behavior
- Deafness
- Does not follow through
- Ear difficulties
- Earaches
- Epilepsy
- Equilibrium
- Excessive talking
- Fatigue
- Feeling closed in
- Frozen feelings
- Hearing difficulties
- Holding back in life
- Infection
- Insanity
- Insomnia
- Internal tension
- Intimidated
- Irritability
- Jaw difficulties
- Joint difficulties
- Lack of discipline
- Lack of spirituality
- Laryngitis
- Loss of memory
- Loss of personal truth
- Low self esteem
- Low self worth
- Motion sickness
- Mouth difficulties
- Multiple Sclerosis
- Neck problems
- Nervous system disorders
- Nervousness
- Neuritis
- Not trusting
- Overly intellectual
- Paralysis
- Parkinson's disease
- Passiveness
- Pridefulness
- Round shoulders
- Self pity
- Sinusitis
- Sore throat
- Speech difficulties
- Sprains
- Stiffness
- Stress
- Throat tightness
- Thyroid difficulties

163

Appendix
One:
Symptoms
and
Imbalances
of the
Chakras

Sixth Chakra Symptoms and Imbalances

- Aging difficulties
- Always has to be the leader
- Amnesia
- Autism
- Birth defects
- Brain tumors
- Caretaker
- Chronic fatigue syndrome
- Coma
- Denies problems
- Depressed
- Does not speak up
- Does not trust
- Does not want to succeed
- Doesn't speak the truth
- Ear infection
- Epilepsy
- Fatigue
- Fevers
- Gray hair
- Growths
- Has all the answers
- Headaches
- Insanity
- Insomnia
- Lack of insight
- Lack of knowledge
- Loss of spiritual connection
- Manipulative
- Memory problems
- Meningitis
- Mental illness
- Migraine headache
- Narcolepsy
- Nervousness
- Not assertive
- Not organized
- Overly intellectual
- Pituitary difficulties
- Quiet
- Retarded
- Schizophrenia
- Senility
- Shy
- Sight
- Sluggish
- Stuck in head
- Sudden energy shifts

Seventh Chakra Symptoms and Imbalances

- Accidents
- Afraid to tap potential
- Aging
- AIDS
- Birth defects
- Brain difficulties
- Cancer of the brain
- Can't concentrate
- Chronic diseases
- Cranial bone difficulties
- Deep depression
- Difficulty making choices
- Does not believe in spirit
- Drug addiction
- Endocrine system difficulties
- Fear of death
- Feeling lost
- Frustration
- Headaches
- Ignorance
- Insanity
- Lack of inspiration
- Living vicariously
- Loss of bliss
- Loss of confidence
- Loss of happiness
- Loss of joy
- Lost interest in life
- Low energy
- Manic-depression
- Nail biting
- Nervousness
- No direction with life
- No enthusiasm
- Not grounded
- Paralysis
- Rebellious
- Seeking acceptance
- Sickly
- Skin growths
- Spaced out
- Suicidal feelings

165

Appendix One: Symptoms and Imbalances of the Chakras

Appendix Two
Emotional Imbalances of the Chakras

1. Emotional imbalances of the first chakra.

The individual is inflexible and unyielding. He is too concerned about survival and security. He does not have the energy to help others. He is self-centered, and places too much importance on the physical world. The individual has a difficult time connecting with spirit.

2. Emotional imbalances of the second chakra.

The individual is overly attached to money, people, places, and things. He is needy and clings to anyone who will listen to him. He is jealous, possessive, and envious of others who have achieved a certain amount of success in their lives. He thinks that material things will bring him happiness.

3. Emotional imbalances of the third chakra.

The individual feels superior to others. He has a strong need to control and dominate others. The person is either quiet and shy, or exploding with anger. The individual likes to dominate others with his superior mental energy. He controls others with his anger and intensity. People are afraid of him, so they do what he wants.

4. Emotional imbalances of the fourth chakra.

The individual feels sad, hurt, or lonely. The person has a difficult time expressing love or being intimate. He is filled with grief and is unable move on with his life in a healthy way. He sees himself as the victim, and looks for sympathy.

5. Emotional imbalances of the fifth chakra.

The person cannot speak the truth. He feels that people will not accept him if he says what is really on his mind. He lies about most things, and does not care who he hurts. He is just concerned with getting his way, and is very self-centered.

6. Emotional imbalances of the sixth chakra.

The individual is afraid of life. He does not have the concentration necessary to complete projects; even taking care of his own personal daily needs becomes tedious. He acts spaced-out and disassociated from life's events. Few things interest him and he can be depressed for long periods of time. He might also hear voices that interfere with his peace of mind.

7. Emotional imbalances of the seventh chakra.

The individual does not feel connected to spirit and wonders why there is so much suffering in this world. He lacks motivation and does not have goals. He seems depressed much of the time and is lethargic. He is disillusioned with the worldly emphasis of acquiring money, but does not know how to break free from this concept. He knows there is something more to life than work, but does not know how to change his thinking and behavior to follow his heart.

Appendix
Two:
Emotional
Imbalances
of the
Chakras

Appendix Three
Meditation
Review

A. Create a meditation space.

B. Set up a prayer table.

C. Light a candle and incense.

D. Begin the meditation with chanting the mantra om three times.

E. Sit quietly on a meditation cushion or pillow for about five minutes and breathe the whole breath. This will quiet your mind and regulate the stress in your body.

F. Determine which chakra is out of balance by using a pendulum or your intuition, or by checking the symptom lists in Appendix One.

G. Use the guided meditations to bring the chakras back into balance.

H. Use the self-help section to follow up with alternative healing modalities to keep the chakras in harmony.

• • •

This process will always keep your chakras in balance and harmony. It is up to you to do the work.

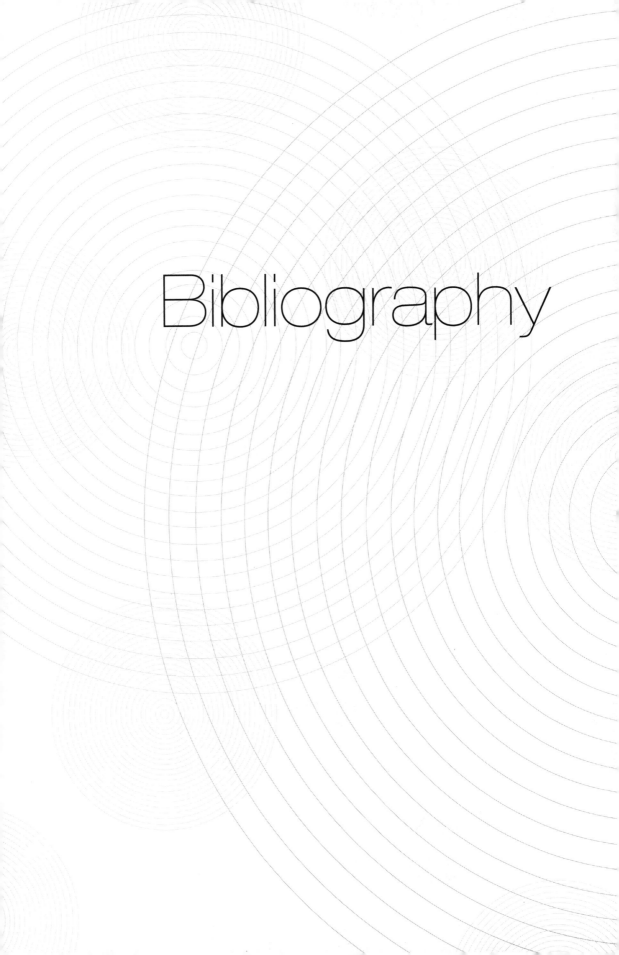

Bibliography

Chakras and Kundalini

Madhusudandasji, Dhyan Yogi Shri, *Shakti: Hidden Treasure of Power*. Clayton, CA: Dhyan Yoga Centers, 1980.

Rhada, Swami Sivananda, *Kundalini: Yoga for the West*. Boulder, CO: Shambhala, 1981.

Rendel, Peter, *Introduction to the Chakras*. New York: Samuel Wiser, 1974.

Anodea, Judith, *Wheels of Life*. St. Paul, MN: Llewellyn Publications, 1988.

Sharma, P.D., *Yoga, Yogasana and Pranayama for Health*. India: Navneet Publications, 1996.

Gardner, Joy, *Color and Crystals: A Journey through the Chakras*. Freedom, CA: The Crossing Press, 1988.

Johari, Harish, *Chakras: Energy Centers of Transformation*. Rochester, Vermont: Destiny Books, 1987

Brennan, Barbara, *Hands of Light*. New York: Bantam Books, 1988.

Mantras

Madhusudandasji, Dhyan Yogi, *Brahmanad: Mantra, Sound and Power*. Clayton, CA: Dhyan Yoga Centers, 1979.

Keshavadas, Satguru Sant, *Healing Techniques of the Holy East*. Oakland, CA: Vishwa Dharma Publishers, 1980.

Radha, Swami Sivananda, *Mantras: Words of Power*. Porthill, ID: Timeless Books, 1980.

Ayurveda

Lad, Vasant, *Ayurveda: The Science of Self-Healing*. Santa Fe, NM: Lotus Press, 1984.

Saraswati, Swami Shivananda, *Yogic Therapy*. Calcutta: Sree Gopal Press, 1985.

Gerson, Scott, Ayurveda: *The Ancient Indian Healing Art*. New York: Barnes and Noble, 1997.

Heyn, Birgit, Ayurveda: *The Indian Art of Natural Medicine and Life Extension*. Rochester, Vermont: Healing Arts Press, 1990.

Swami, Abhedananda, *The Yoga Psychology*. Hollywood: Vedanta Press, 1967.

Subramuniyaswami, Sivaya, *Dancing With Siva*. Concord, CA: Himalayan Academy, 1993.

Ramacharaka, Yogi, *Hatha Yoga*. Chicago: Yogi Publication Society, 1990.

Diet

Airola, Pavvo, *Are You Confused?* Phoenix: Health Plus, 1971.

Ballentine, Rudolph, *Diet and Nutrition*. Honesdale, PA: Himalayan International Institute, 1978.

Nelson, Dennis, *Food Combining Simplified*. Santa Cruz, CA: The Plan, 1985.

Homeopathy

Dancu, David, *Homeopathic Vibrations*. Boulder, CO: Sunshine Press, 1996.

Panos, Maesimund and Jane Heimlich, *Homeopathic Medicine at Home*. New York: The Putnam Publishing Group, 1976.

Herbs

Kloss, Jethro, *Back to Eden*. Loma Linda, CA: Back to Eden Publishing Company, 1992.

Tierra, Michael, *The Way of Herbs*. New York: Simon and Schuster, 1990.

Affirmations

Hartzell, Shanta, *Angel Messages*. Kaneohe, Hawaii: Angelic Dimensions Publishing, 1997.

Hay, Louise, *Heal Yourself*. Los Angeles: Hay House, 1997.

Other books by Maruti Seidman

A Guide to Polarity Therapy: The Gentle Art of Hands on Healing

• • •

Polarity Balancing Certification Program

Maruti Seidman has been teaching and certifying practitioners in his basic 120-hour Polarity Balancing Certification Program since 1980. He has taught at many of the leading Massage Schools and Centers throughout the United States.

• • •

The Chakra Awareness Workshop

Maruti Seidman has developed The Chakra Awareness Workshop. This class is designed to assist the individual in experiencing and healing their Chakra System.

• • •

If you would like more information about Maruti Seidman and his programs and schedule, or want him to come to your community to teach, please write to him at P.O. Box 3175, Boulder, Colorado 80307 or call toll free, 1 (800) 334-4097 or (303) 499-5198.

Oh Heavenly Father

Oh Heavenly Father
We thank you for your blessings
And the strength you give us.
Your love vibrations unite the entire
Universe and all its life forms.
We are just a reflection of you—
Glowing, shining, and full of light.
The only peace we know is the peace
You give us. The only happiness we
Know is the happiness you give us.
The only bliss we know is the bliss
You give us. We are blessed by your
Essence, and will always be humbly
At your feet.